USMLE Step 2

The Stanford Solutions

To the NBME Computer-Based
Sample Test Questions

Written by

The Stanford Solutions Team

Scott J. Kush
Stanford School of Medicine, Class of 2002

Tessa L. Walters
Stanford School of Medicine
Class of 1999

Devon J. Webster
Stanford School of Medicine
Class of 1999

Roni Zeiger
Stanford School of Medicine
Class of 1999

Niaz Banaiee
Stanford School of Medicine
Class of 2001

Lisa Ann Carroll
Stanford School of Medicine
Class of 2001

Swaine L. Chen
Stanford School of Medicine
Class of 2003

Sujoya Dey
Stanford School of Medicine
Class of 2000

Amarjit Dosanjh
Stanford School of Medicine
Class of 2002

Shireen Victoria Guide
Stanford School of Medicine
Class of 2000

George R. Matcuk Jr.
Stanford School of Medicine
Class of 2003

Saman Nazarian
Stanford School of Medicine
Class of 1999

Mychelle L. Shegog
Stanford School of Medicine
Class of 2001

Planet Med Publishing
PO BOX 3053
Stanford, CA 94309

Planet Med

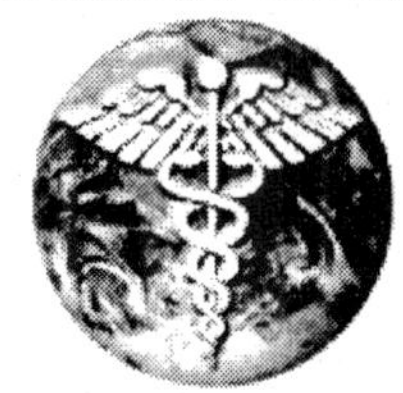

Publishing

http://www.planetusmle.com

Cover Design: George R. Matcuk Jr.

ISBN: 1-893730-25-5

Printed in the United States of America

Editor

Tessa L. Walters

Faculty Reviewers

James W. Chu, MD
Postdoctoral Fellow
Division of Endocrinology
Department of Medicine
Stanford University School of Medicine

Harcharan P. S. Gill, MD
Associate Professor
Department of Urology
Stanford University School of Medicine

Bertil E. Glader, MD PhD
Professor
Division of Hematology and Oncology
Department of Pediatrics
Stanford University School of Medicine

Edward D. Harris Jr., MD
Professor,
Division of Immunology and
Rheumatology
Department of Medicine
Stanford University School of Medicine

Phillip M. Harter, MD FACEP
Clinical Associate Professor
Associate Residency Program Director
Division of Emergency Medicine
Department of Surgery
Stanford University School of Medicine

R. Harold Holbrook Jr., MD
Associate Professor
Division of Maternal-Fetal Medicine
Department of
Gynecology and Obstetrics
Stanford University School of Medicine

Charlotte D. Jacobs, MD
Professor
Director, Clinical Cancer Center
Division of Oncology
Department of Medicine
Stanford University School of Medicine

Samuel LeBaron, MD PhD
Associate Professor
Division of Family
and Community Medicine
Department of Medicine
Stanford University School of Medicine

Carrie W. Loutit, MD
Staff Physician
Department of Pediatrics
Stanford University School of Medicine

Jeffery S. Loutit, MBBCh
Chief of Infectious Diseases
Palo Alto VA Health Care System
Assistant Professor of Medicine
Division of Infectious Disease
Stanford University School of Medicine

Lawrence H. Mathers Jr., MD PhD
Associate Professor of
Pediatrics and Anatomy
Chief, Division of Human Anatomy
Stanford University School of Medicine

Lars Osterberg, MD
Staff Physician
Palo Alto Veterans Affairs Hospital
Department of Internal Medicine
Stanford University School of Medicine

Julie Parsonnet, MD
Associate Professor
Division of Infectious Diseases
Department of Medicine
Division of Epidemiology
Department of Health Research and Policy
Stanford University School of Medicine

Klaus J. Porzig, MD
Clinical Professor
Department of Medicine
Stanford University School of Medicine

Adam Seiver, MD
Clinical Assistant Professor
Division of Trauma & Surgical Critical Care
Department of Surgery
Stanford University School of Medicine

David Lawrence Smith, MD
Staff Psychiatrist
and Research Fellow
Department of Psychiatry
Stanford University School of Medicine

Jon C. Starr, MD
Assistant Professor
Director, Division of Dermatologic Surgery
Department of Dermatology
Stanford University School of Medicine

Elliott Wolfe, MD FACP
Associate Dean for Student Affairs
Clinical Professor of Medicine
Stanford University School of Medicine

Student Reviewers

Helen Deng
Sharon K. Dhanowa
Lan Hue Ly
Jonathan A. Mathy
Svetlana A. Pilyugina
Jacqueline Nerney Welch

Dedicated To:

The Students

of

Stanford University School of Medicine

Thanks for making medical school less about competition and more about collaboration, cooperation, and camaraderie.

- The Stanford Solutions Team

Foreword

After years of clinical practice and teaching, I learned a powerful formula about the practice of medicine: **Knowledge + Experience = Competence + Confidence.** *Knowledge* of the science of medicine begins in medical school. *Experience* begins in the clinical years and excitement is often an emotional companion. In my third-year, on an internal medicine clerkship, a resident assigned me to a new patient. The patient had presented with chest pain and the resident had given an initial diagnosis of unstable angina. At the bedside it was apparent there was a pleuritic component to the pain; a careful examination disclosed a three-component cardiac sound – one I had never heard before. I surmised it was a pericardial friction rub and the patient's problem was acute pericarditis not ischemic heart disease! With each passing clerkship I became expert at cardiac auscultation. *Experience* also leads to professional clinical judgment and the formula for the practice of medicine finally matures to encompass *Competence* and *Confidence.*

During the fourth month of my internship year my resident, Alan, called with information about our next admission: a patient with upper gastrointestinal hemorrhage. When the patient arrived, it became clear that nausea with repeated retching had caused minor bleeding – finding the reason for the nausea would be the key to the diagnosis. My physical examination disclosed evidence of dehydration. As I drew my first tube of blood I immediately noticed the peculiar color of the venous blood; it appeared as if milk and blood had been churned together! It was my first experience with severe hyperlipemia in the setting of diabetic ketoacidosis; the hyperlipemia was visible in the retina (lipemia retinalis) as well. When I told Alan about my diagnosis he shouted "hooray" and praised my achievement; I frequently remember the *Confidence* and excitement I felt at having achieved a new level of clinical *Competence.*

Upon arrival, USMLE Step 2 rests waiting to test new clinicians on the first two milestones: *Knowledge* and (early) *Experience. The Stanford Solutions* provides accurate, expanded answers – with supportive information – to the USMLE sample practice questions provided by the National Board of Medical Examiners. These cogent elaborations provide waves of information extending from each question's core. The knowledge and energy of Stanford's faculty and students are combined in *The Stanford Solutions* to assist with your USMLE passage to residency and ultimately in increasing your *Competence* and *Confidence.*

Elliott Wolfe, MD FACP
Associate Dean
Stanford University School of Medicine

Introduction

It amazes me how fast time flies. And now, it is about to move even faster as we've just launched directly into the digital age. Even the boards exam, which for decades was done with pencil and paper, will now be a series of ones and zeroes.

The recent change to computer-based testing is a big one. Medical students will now want to become as familiar as possible with the new testing interface. Some students will initially fear this new way of taking tests, while others will approach it like seasoned pros. Probably the best advice is to just sit back, relax, and simply realize that, independent of the new format, this is still just a test.

One thing is for certain, it always helps to look at sample questions from the source. For the boards, and specifically the Step 1 exam, this means reading *NBME's Computer-Based Sample Questions.* These questions are readily available, as every student should receive these questions in a booklet with their Step 2 registration materials.

Introduced for this year is a whole new set of sample questions. These questions are an effort by the NBME to assist you in getting a sense of the type of material you'll likely be asked on the exam. You would have to be crazy to skip over these questions. They are *straight from the source*, and therefore are the purest facsimile of the actual exam.

Additionally, students receive these very same questions on a CD-ROM as a way to try out the new testing format. DON'T WAIT to try out the CD-ROM. You should become as well acquainted with the new testing interface as possible. You will want to be able to transition easily from one question to another, and from one window to another, without hesitation. Only by becoming completely "at home" with the new interface will your test day go as smoothly as you imagine.

To assist you in preparing for this new exam, we have undertaken the mammoth task of finding the solutions to all 150 computer-based sample questions. We go well beyond the simple one-letter answer you're initially provided, and provide full descriptions of the right answer as well as explanations of the wrong answers. We think you'll find our answers very comprehensive and well researched.

While working on this task, we learned that no one individual could have ever taken on a task this large (and still be sane), but that as a team we were able to provide the VERY BEST answers possible.

We hope you'll learn a tremendous amount of relevant information from these solutions (we sure did). We also hope that it proves to be one of your most valuable study aids for your upcoming exam.

Enjoy your journey through *The Stanford Solutions*, and good luck!

Scott J. Kush
October, 1999
Stanford, CA

WANT TO CONTRIBUTE?
Did you find an error?
Tell us!

(If we use it, we'll acknowledge you in future editions.)

Send e-mail to: skush@planetusmle.com

Or visit

THE CENTER OF THE UNIVERSE

www.PlanetUSMLE.com

(you will also find updates to our book on the website)

Guide To Using The Stanford Solutions

By now you probably have received a publication by the National Board of Medical Examiners entitled *Step 2: Computer-Based Content and Sample Test Questions.* This publication is typically available from your medical school's student affairs office. And now, everything is also available via the USMLE website (http://www.usmle.org/). In the booklet (or digital version), you will find 150 sample questions that give you a great example of what questions will be like on the computer-based USMLE Step 2 exam. Along with the booklet, you should have also received a companion CD-ROM containing the same questions found in the booklet but in actual exam simulation format. The program on the CD-ROM is also available for download from the USMLE website.

Now assuming that you have the questions, you should find the following 150 solutions to be clear, straightforward and comprehensive. After reading a given solution, you should easily be able to determine why a given answer is correct and why all others are incorrect.

In every case, the important learning points are emphasized in our answers so that you won't be confused or frustrated by the question. It is important for you to know that for one question in this book, we have found that our solution has led us to a different answer than what the NBME suggests. In that case I can confidently state that we have double-checked with our faculty reviewers and stand strongly by our answer. It is likely that the NBME will in the future fix this error and even possibly change the question. In any case, we have flagged this question for you.

We invite you to check our website where updates to the book will periodically be made available to solve general ambiguities and potentially resolve any future changes to the questions by the NBME. If you find you can make a contribution to our answers or can correct an error in our work, please send us an e-mail and we'll include your contribution in the next edition.

We know that studying for the boards can, at times, be very overwhelming. In an effort to make this task less daunting, the solutions have been written to focus in on the most important information. We have also tried to add a bit of humor in these answers to make your travels a bit more interesting. We sincerely hope that these solutions help you in your journey. Good luck on the boards!

www.PlanetUSMLE.com

The Stanford Solutions

1

(Block 1: Item 1)

(E)

In a case-control (or retrospective) study, subjects are chosen based on the presence of disease, and historical information is gathered retrospectively to attempt to identify risk factors for the disease. In contrast, in a cohort, or prospective, study, subjects are chosen based on the presence of risk factors, and subjects are followed over time to see if they develop disease. Generally, cohort studies are better than case-control studies at establishing the risk factors that cause disease, because case-control studies have several possible biases. (Note that both cohort and case-control studies are observational, and so neither are as powerful as experimental studies.) Because case-control studies frequently rely on people's memory, they are subject to **recall bias**. Recall bias means that subjects whose lives have been affected by disease may recall events or exposures differently than control subjects.

Because risk (cumulative incidence) in exposed and in unexposed individuals cannot be calculated in a case-control study, risk ratios (frequently termed relative risk) comparing exposed and unexposed cannot be calculated. An odds ratio is a good estimate of relative risk unless the risk factor of interest is very common. An odds ratio is the odds of exposure among cases divided by the odds of exposure among controls.

Statistical power is the probability that a study will detect a difference between groups if the difference really exists. If a statistically significant difference is found, then power is adequate. If no difference is found, then we have to wonder if there is truly no difference, or if the power was not adequate to demonstrate it. A study is considered **statistically significant** if the 95% confidence interval of the relative risk does not include 1.0. If it does, then you cannot be 95% sure that the relative risk is not 1.0, which would mean that subjects and controls are equally likely to have disease. A "p value" of less than 0.05 demonstrates the same statistical significance by showing that there is less than a 5% chance that this difference occurred by chance alone. There are no issues of **diagnostic bias** or **ecologic fallacy** in this question.

Dawson-Saunders, 2nd ed., pp 7-17, 55, 95, 170, 273-74.

2

(Block 1: Item 2)

(D)

Classic symptoms and signs of chronic obstructive pulmonary disease (COPD) include dyspnea on exertion, cough, increased anteroposterior chest diameter ("barrel chested"), increased resonance on percussion, and end-expiratory wheezes. The **influenza A vaccine** should be given annually to the following groups: healthy adults older than age 65; anyone with chronic cardiopulmonary disease (e.g., COPD), metabolic or renal disease, or hemoglobinopathy; anyone taking immunosuppressive drugs; health care workers; nursing home residents; and anyone who has contact with the above-mentioned at-risk groups.

After receiving the primary series of immunizations against tetanus and diphtheria, it is recommended that adults receive a **tetanus and diphtheria booster (Td)** every ten years. The ***Hemophilus influenzae*** **Type b ("Hib") vaccine** is recommended for all children, as well as those adults who have sickle cell disease, are asplenic, transplant recipients, or are receiving certain types of chemotherapy. The recombinant **hepatitis B vaccine** series is recommended for intravenous drug users, male homosexuals, sexual contacts of hepatitis B carriers, and health care workers. It is also required for all school children in California. The **pneumococcal vaccine** contains polysaccharides from the capsule of the 23 most common strains of *Streptococcus pneumoniae*. It is recommended for healthy adults over 65 years old, those without a spleen, persons with sickle cell disease, chronic cardiopulmonary disease (e.g., COPD), cirrhosis, alcoholics, and the immunocompromised. A single dose usually results in life-long immunity, but revaccination every 6 years should be considered in asplenic and other high-risk patients (remember that the spleen is the key defense against encapsulated organisms such as *Streptococcus pneumoniae*, *Hemophilus influenzae*, and *Neisseria meningitidis*).

Adults (over 25 years old) should also receive one dose of the measles vaccine if they were born in 1957 or later (health care workers, college students, and travelers should receive two doses) and the rubella vaccine if they were born after 1956. Adults aged 25-64 years should also receive the mumps vaccine. CDC recommendations suggest polio vaccination for the following high-risk adults: travelers to countries where poliomyelitis is epidemic or endemic, people who live in communities with disease caused by wild type polio, lab workers and health care workers who may have contact with polioviruses, and unvaccinated adults whose children will be receiving OPV (oral live vaccine). Hepatitis A vaccine is recommended for travelers to countries with endemic infection, homosexual males, illegal drug users, people with chronic liver disease or clotting factor disorders, and possibly food handlers. Varicella vaccine is indicated for people with no history of varicella disease (e.g., chickenpox) or vaccination. It is also indicated for those that are seronegative, susceptible health care workers, susceptible contacts of immunocompromised people, and susceptible people who are at high risk of exposure (remember, varicella vaccine is contraindicated during pregnancy).

Fauci, 14th ed., pp 538, 649, 845.
Tierney, 38th ed., pp 1217-24.
http://www.cdc.gov/nip/schedule/adult/

3

(Block 1: Item 3)

(E)

Mid-line chest pain that is aggravated by spicy foods is often due to gastroesophageal reflux disease (GERD), or "heartburn," which refers to the symptoms caused by reflux of gastric contents into the esophagus. However, bending or lying down typically exacerbates GERD, and H2-receptor blockers usually provide some relief of symptoms. This type of chest pain in a patient with AIDS, or any other condition leading to an immunosuppressed state, leads one to be concerned about infectious esophagitis. Common etiologies include *Candida albicans*, herpes simplex virus (HSV), and cytomegalovirus (CMV). Typical symptoms are odynophagia (sharp substernal pain on swallowing) and dysphagia (difficulty with swallowing). Most patients with esophageal candidiasis also have oral candidiasis (thrush). Patients with HSV esophagitis may have oral herpes simplex ulcers, and those with CMV esophagitis may have colonic or retinal CMV infection. Oral candida in an immunosuppressed patient can progress to involve the esophagus. Although clotrimazole troches (lozenges) are generally effective against thrush, topical therapy is not usually effective against candidal esophagitis in immunocompromised patients. Instead, initial therapy is with oral fluconazole, and intravenous amphotericin is used for those not responding to oral therapy. Suspected candidal esophagitis is generally treated empirically with fluconazole. In order to evaluate the possibility of HSV or CMV esophagitis, **esophagoscopy** is reserved for those who do not improve. If HSV esophagitis is suspected (e.g., the patient has oral ulcers), a **therapeutic trial of acyclovir** would be reasonable. However, a definitive diagnosis can be made by esophagoscopy—yellow-white plaques on the mucosa characterize candidal esophagitis, a few large, shallow ulcerations typify CMV esophagitis, and multiple small, deep ulcerations characterize HSV esophagitis. CMV esophagitis is treated with intravenous ganciclovir or foscarnet. Immune-competent patients with herpes esophagitis are treated symptomatically, while those who are immunosuppressed are given oral or intravenous acyclovir.

Esophagoscopy, or upper endoscopy, is the best study for evaluating persistent heartburn or odynophagia. A **portable pH probe** can also be placed in the esophagus to monitor the acidity in the esophagus and determine if symptoms correspond to documented reflux. This can be useful to confirm the diagnosis of GERD in a patient that is not responding to treatment. The **acid perfusion test** has been used to diagnose esophagitis. Hydrochloric acid is delivered through a nasoesophageal tube, alternating with saline. If pain occurs in response to acid perfusion and not in response to saline, the test is considered positive for esophagitis. Not surprisingly, the acid perfusion test has been used less frequently since the advent of endoscopy and ambulatory pH monitoring. **Esophageal manometry** (a procedure in which a catheter is placed in the esophagus to measure pressure) is the ideal way to study esophageal motility. This should be done to evaluate dysphagia after esophagoscopy or barium swallow studies have ruled out a mechanical cause. Manometry can measure the waves of peristalsis in the esophagus and the pressures at the upper and lower esophageal sphincters. In addition to evaluating motility disorders, esophageal manometry can demonstrate decreased pressure at the lower esophageal sphincter that can allow reflux of stomach contents and cause GERD.

Fauci, 14th ed., pp 1589-90.
Tierney, 38th ed., pp 283, 563-64, 568-69, 1237.

4

(Block 1: Item 4)

(C)

"Stroke" refers to the abrupt onset of focal neurological deficits. Strokes are generally subdivided into two main categories: ischemic (which can be thrombotic or embolic) and hemorrhagic. Stroke is also used more specifically to mean cerebral infarction, or death of neurological tissue due to ischemia. If cerebral ischemia lasts more than a few minutes, infarction of brain tissue occurs. A transient ischemic attack (TIA) can cause the same neurological deficits, but unlike a stroke it resolves completely within 24 hours (usually within a few hours) because it does not cause infarction. Although this patient seems to have only hemisensory loss and hemiparesis, carotid circulation lesions can also produce homonymous hemianopsia, ipsilateral monocular visual loss (amaurosis fugax), dysarthria, and aphasia.

The most common causes of cerebral ischemia and infarction are atherosclerosis with thromboembolism (such as an atherosclerotic plaque from the carotid artery embolizing to the brain) and cardiogenic embolism (when a piece of thrombus in a heart chamber embolizes to the brain). Risk factors for stroke include hypertension, diabetes, hyperlipidemia, smoking, heart disease, heavy alcohol use, cocaine use, and family history of stroke. The neurological deficits depend on the vessels involved. [A quick review: the anterior cerebral artery (ACA) and middle cerebral artery (MCA) are derived from the internal carotid artery, while the posterior cerebral artery is the extension of the vertebral arteries (the so-called "posterior circulation").] Infarcts involving the ACA and MCA typically cause contralateral hemiplegia and hemianesthesia. Because the ACA supplies the medial portions of the hemispheres, the hemiplegia seen when it is infarcted usually involves the lower extremities. Since the MCA supplies the lateral hemispheres, its infarction typically causes a hemiplegia involving the arms and face. To remember which part of the cortex controls which part of the body, think of the homunculus tripping on the falx cerebri and doing a face-plant on the parietal lobe while his foot gets stuck in between the hemispheres. Ischemia or infarction of the posterior circulation classically causes ipsilateral cranial nerve deficits, ataxia (secondary to cerebellar infarct), and contralateral sensory or motor deficits.

The treatment of stroke depends on its etiology and time course. If a stroke is worsening, anticoagulation with heparin may limit its progression. If a stroke patient is able to get to the hospital within 3 hours of symptom onset, intravenous thrombolytic therapy with tissue plasminogen activator (t-PA) can reduce the neurological deficit. t-PA has not been shown to be safe or effective after 3 hours has passed from the initial onset of symptoms. Prior to anticoagulation or thrombolytic therapy, a **head CT scan** should be performed to rule out intracranial bleeding. Bleeding may be present at the site of an ischemic stroke, or the stroke may be a hemorrhagic stroke instead of an ischemic stroke. Hemorrhagic strokes include subarachnoid hemorrhage that is usually due to ruptured aneurysms or arteriovenous malformations, and intracerebral hemorrhage that is usually secondary to hypertension. In addition, a patient with stroke may also fall and develop an epidural or subdural hematoma. Evidence of intracranial bleeding is an absolute contraindication for the administration of anticoagulants or thrombolytics.

The evaluation of a stroke is directed at finding the cause. A bruit heard over the carotid artery suggests that a plaque there could be an embolic source (but carotid bruits alone are an unreliable indicator of clinically significant atherosclerosis). After immediate therapy such as heparin or t-PA, if indicated, ultrasound with Doppler **(a carotid duplex scan)** is used to identify and quantify a stenosis of the internal carotid artery. However, ultrasound cannot distinguish between near-complete and complete carotid occlusion. **Carotid angiography** is needed to make this important distinction (which may affect whether or not a patient should undergo a corrective surgery—carotid endarterectomy). If a stroke patient has a heart murmur or if heart disease is suspected, an ECG should be done to look for evidence of an arrhythmia (e.g. atrial fibrillation) that may have dislodged a piece of thrombus or a recent myocardial infarction that could have predisposed to thrombus formation. **Echocardiography** should also be performed to look for a thrombus in the heart. If a thrombus is found, the patient should begin chronic anticoagulation therapy. **Electroencephalography** (EEG) is not useful in the evaluation of stroke, but rather in the evaluation of seizure. However, it is not always possible to distinguish a TIA from a seizure, and EEG may help in such a situation.

Fauci, 14th ed., pp 2325, 2334-35.
Ferri, 3rd ed., pp 674-89.
Tierney, 38th ed., pp 943-49.

5

(Block 1: Item 5)

(A)

Pelvic inflammatory disease (PID) is generally considered an infection of the fallopian tubes, but it can affect the uterus and ovaries as well. It is typically polymicrobial, and is associated with the sexually transmitted organisms *Neisseria gonorrhea* and *Chlamydia trachomatis*, as well as with members of the vaginal flora such as *Gardnerella vaginalis*, *Hemophilus influenzae* and enteric Gram-negative rods. It is thought that invading bacteria such as *N. gonorrhea* and *C. trachomatis* change the local environment to allow normally non-pathogenic bacteria to thrive. PID typically occurs in young women with multiple sexual partners. Symptoms and signs can be very subtle but include lower abdominal pain, fevers and chills, irregular vaginal bleeding, purulent cervical discharge, cervical motion tenderness, and adnexal tenderness. Right upper quadrant pain may be present if there is an associated perihepatitis (Fitz-Hugh-Curtis syndrome). PID can even present as peritonitis and septic shock. There may be an elevated white blood cell count, but this is neither sensitive nor specific.

Because the presentation can be subtle and non-specific, it is often difficult to distinguish PID from other conditions such as appendicitis and ectopic pregnancy. The diagnosis of PID is more certain if culture of the cervical discharge grows *N. gonorrhea* or *C. trachomatis*, but action must be taken before these results are available. A quantitative serum β-hCG (human chorionic gonadotropin) should be obtained, since in an ectopic pregnancy the levels will be higher than in a non-pregnant female but lower than in a normal pregnancy of the same gestational age. Pelvic or vaginal ultrasound can help identify an ectopic pregnancy older than 6 weeks. Appendicitis classically causes right lower quadrant pain and is not associated with cervical exudate. Laparoscopy with visualization of the fallopian tubes is the only reliable method of diagnosing PID. Laparoscopy should be performed if the diagnosis is in doubt or the patient has not improved with 48 hours of antibiotic therapy. **Antibiotics** should be started immediately to prevent the long-term sequelae of PID, which include chronic abdominal pain, infertility, and ectopic pregnancy. These complications result from scarring of the fallopian tubes. Antibiotics must cover the broad spectrum of organisms that can cause PID. A recommended outpatient regimen is ofloxacin (covers *N. gonorrhea*, *C. trachomatis*, and Gram-negative rods) and metronidazole (covers anaerobes). Hospitalization is recommended for patients with peritonitis, high fever, inability to take oral antibiotics, ectopic pregnancy, or suspected pelvic abscess, or if **appendicitis** cannot be ruled out.

Culdocentesis is a needle aspiration of intraperitoneal fluid or blood through a puncture of the posterior vaginal fornix into the cul-de-sac. It can help distinguish an ectopic pregnancy or hemorrhagic ovarian cyst from a ruptured pelvic abscess or ruptured appendix. The former would lead to blood in the peritoneum, whereas in the later, pus would be found in the peritoneum. A Meckel's diverticulum is formed when a small portion of the embryonic vitelline duct persists and forms an outpouching of the ileum. It is the most common congenital gastrointestinal anomaly, and though rarely symptomatic after age five, it can present with bleeding, small bowel obstruction, or inflammation in young adults. Inflammation of the diverticulum can mimic appendicitis. A Meckel's diverticulum can often be diagnosed with a **Meckel's scan** in which an isotope scan of the abdomen is performed after injecting technetium intravenously. The technetium is taken up by ectopic gastric mucosa that is often found in these diverticula. A **dilation and curettage** ("D & C") consists of dilating the neck of the uterus and scraping off a sample of its lining, the endometrium. It is most commonly performed to remove products of conception, or to obtain a histological sample of the endometrium to evaluate disorders such as irregular vaginal bleeding.

Benson, 3rd ed., pp 170-73.
Fauci, 14th ed., p 1648.
Tierney, 38th ed., pp 716-17.

6

(Block 1: Item 6)

(C)

Delirium is an acute confusional state in which consciousness (awareness) is impaired. It is frequently contrasted with dementia, which has a chronic onset and is characterized by diminished mental function (particularly diminished memory). Delirium has an extensive differential diagnosis including: drugs—anticholinergics, narcotics, and steroids; systemic problems—infection and hypoxemia; metabolic disorders—liver failure, hypo/hyper-glycemia; and electrolyte imbalances—hypo/hyper-natremia, and hypo/hyper-calcemia. Urinary tract infections can commonly cause delirium, especially in older patients, with or without pyelonephritis. Pyelonephritis classically presents with fever, shaking chills, nausea, symptoms of lower urinary tract infection (UTI: urinary frequency, urgency, and dysuria), and costovertebral angle tenderness. Complete blood count reveals an increased white blood cell (WBC) count. Urinalysis demonstrates bacteria, elevated WBC (≥ 5 WBC per high power field), and may show white cell casts and mild proteinuria.

Pyelonephritis usually begins as a lower UTI and ascends to the kidneys via the ureters. Colonic bacteria are the typical infective agents, with ***Escherichia coli*** being by far the most common. While the majority of these agents are gram negative rods (GNR), gram positive bacteria such as *Enterococcus* could also be involved and thus initial antibiotic coverage should include both GNR and gram positive coverage. *Proteus*, *Klebsiella*, and *Enterobacter* are less common culprits in uncomplicated infections (that is, in patients without urological abnormalities or urinary catheters). The above GNRs plus ***Pseudomonas*** and *Serratia* are common causes of UTI in patients with catheters, in patients status-post urologic manipulation, and in hospitalized patients. *Staphylococcus saprophyticus* is a common cause of UTI in young women. ***Staphylococcus aureus*** typically reaches the kidneys via the hematogenous route, usually from a source outside the urinary tract such as an abscess. In addition, *S. aureus* is more commonly associated with UTI in patients with renal stones or previous urological instrumentation. Pyelonephritis, regardless of the causative agent, can lead to bacteremia if the infection spreads from the kidney to the bloodstream. Bacteremia means that there are bacteria in the blood, as shown by a positive blood culture, while septic shock refers to the life-threatening systemic manifestations of infection that can be due to bacterial cell wall components. Septic shock is usually due to Gram-negative rod bacteremia, but it can also occur with Gram-positive cocci (Staphylococcus and **Streptococcus**) and Gram-negative anaerobes (e.g., ***Bacteroides fragilis***). Signs of septic shock include hypotension, tachycardia, hyperventilation, cold extremities, renal failure (decreased urine output and elevated serum creatinine) and altered mental status.

Candida and other fungi commonly colonize the urine of catheterized patients and diabetics, and may ascend to the kidney; they can then invade the bloodstream and seed other areas such as the retina, brain, and myocardium. ***Bacteroides fragilis*** is an anaerobic Gram-negative rod that is part of the normal bowel flora. It typically forms abscesses, and can rarely cause a renal abscess secondary to *Bacteroides* bacteremia. ***Streptococcus pyogenes* (group A Strep)** is the most common bacterial cause of sore throat with scarlet fever and rheumatic fever as possible sequelae. Group A Strep also causes cellulitis, impetigo, erysipelas, lymphangitis, and bacteremia by traversing skin defects. After delivery, it can cause endometritis and sepsis (puerperal fever).

Fauci, 14th ed., pp 818, 992.
Ferri, 3rd ed., pp 162-64, 557-60.
Nicoll, 2nd ed., pp 231, 364.
Tierney, 38th ed., pp 482, 1042, 1419.

7

(Block 1: Item 7)

(D)

Abnormal vaginal bleeding is a common presenting symptom. If this occurs in a woman in her reproductive years, the first step is to rule out pregnancy, since miscarriage and ectopic pregnancy can cause bleeding. With a negative pregnancy test, major causes of irregular vaginal bleeding should be considered: anovulation (break through bleeding), benign growths such as uterine fibroids and uterine or cervical polyps, cervical cancer and endometrial hyperplasia or endometrial cancer. Another common cause of chronic anovulatory bleeding in women of reproductive age is polycystic ovary syndrome, which is associated with infertility, hirsutism, and obesity.

Because endometrial cancer is uncommon in women younger than 40, women in this age group with a normal physical exam and Pap smear can be given a trial of oral contraceptives, which can normalize anovulatory bleeding. However, continued irregular bleeding does merit an endometrial biopsy. If the woman is over age 40 or post-menopausal, an **endometrial biopsy** is a priority to rule out uterine malignancy. Although uterine fibroids still account for most cases of abnormal bleeding in this older group, endometrial carcinoma accounts for up to 25% of cases and should be diagnosed as promptly as possible. It is the most common female genital cancer, with a peak incidence between the ages of 55 and 60. Risk factors include obesity, nulliparity, late menopause, and chronic unopposed estrogen stimulation of the uterus. Because of this last risk factor, **estrogen replacement therapy (ERT)** for postmenopausal women, which has been shown to decrease osteoporosis and cardiovascular disease, is now given in conjunction with progesterone. Women without a uterus may receive unopposed estrogen. Endometrial carcinoma may present with only vaginal bleeding, though a pelvic mass is sometimes found on pelvic exam. If endometrial biopsy provides an adequate sample and there is no evidence of malignancy, a post-menopausal woman with irregular bleeding may be started on hormone replacement therapy to normalize the bleeding.

Other common causes of abnormal vaginal bleeding in post-menopausal women are atrophic vaginitis, cervical polyps, and uterine prolapse. Atrophic vaginitis is more common in those who have not received ERT since the vaginal mucosa atrophies in the absence of estrogen. Atrophic vaginitis and uterine prolapse are apparent on pelvic exam, while a cervical polyp is only visible if it is near the cervical os. Cervical carcinoma is uncommon in women over age 55 who have had normal Pap smears regularly.

As mentioned above, women younger than 40 with normal pelvic exam and Pap smear can be given a trial of oral contraceptives to normalize irregular vaginal bleeding. These contraceptives should contain both estrogen and progesterone, since unopposed estrogen can lead to endometrial hyperplasia (and therefore cause additional irregular bleeding!). If an informative sample is not obtained by endometrial biopsy, a dilation and curettage ("D & C") with hysteroscopy should be considered. The D & C obtains much more endometrial tissue for histological examination than does an endometrial biopsy, and hysteroscopy allows for direct visualization of possible growths in the uterus. Women with no evidence of malignancy and normal anatomy by hysteroscopy may benefit from **ablation of the endometrium**, in which the surface of the endometrium is destroyed with electrocautery or photocoagulation. The purpose of ablation is to reduce or prevent future menstrual flow by destroying the tissue that normally bleeds (therefore, it should not be done on women who may want to become pregnant in the future). There is often a reduction in PMS symptoms as well. **Colposcopy** is a low-power magnification exam of the cervix after applying 5% acetic acid (vinegar) to its surface. Its purpose is to identify areas of pre-cancer or cancer in the area of the cervix where cancer most frequently develops, the transformation zone (where the transition occurs from columnar epithelium of the uterus to squamous epithelium of the vagina). The acetic acid makes abnormal areas turn white ("aceto-whitening") so they are easier seen and biopsied. Colposcopy is performed on any patient with a Pap smear suggestive of malignancy.

Benson, 1st ed., pp 29-31, 200-01.
Goroll, 3rd ed., pp 597-601, 649.

8

(Block 1: Item 8)

(B)

Low hematocrit, hypotension, tachycardia, and oliguria on postoperative day 1 in a patient status-post ruptured aortic aneurysm repair are highly suspicious for acute blood loss. An unfortunate sequela of **hypovolemia** is prerenal failure, manifest as oliguria, diffuse peripheral edema and low urine sodium.

Acute renal failure (ARF) is a sudden decrease in renal function. Increased serum creatinine is a useful marker for renal failure. Creatinine typically doubles each time the glomerular filtration rate (GFR) decreases by 50%. ARF is often accompanied by oliguria, which is defined by a urine output of < 500 mL per day, or < 20 mL per hour. Symptoms that are due to uremia (the accumulation of nitrogenous wastes, also known as azotemia) include nausea, vomiting, and altered mental status. Other symptoms and signs depend on the etiology of the renal failure, which can be classified as prerenal, intrinsic, or postrenal failure. In prerenal failure, the kidneys are subject to inadequate blood flow, as occurs in hypovolemia or low cardiac output. Hypovolemia may be due to poor volume intake, overuse of diuretics, or blood loss such as from gastrointestinal losses or an internal hemorrhage. Low cardiac output can result from **congestive heart failure** (CHF), cardiogenic shock, or a pulmonary embolus. A patient in CHF will likely have pulmonary edema, distended neck veins, and an extra heart sound (S_3). Signs of hypovolemia include hypotension and tachycardia.

Intrinsic renal failure results from dysfunction of the renal tubules, interstitium, vasculature, or glomeruli. There are three main categories of intrinsic renal failure: (1) acute tubular necrosis (ATN) which can be caused by ischemia (and can follow prerenal failure) or nephrotoxic drugs such as aminoglycosides and radiographic contrast media; (2) interstitial nephritis, which is usually a allergic reaction to drugs such as penicillins, cephalosporins, sulfonamides, and NSAIDs; and (3) glomerulonephritis, as in post-streptococcal or lupus glomerulonephritis. Postrenal failure is usually the easiest to exclude. It results from obstruction of the urinary tract such as by stones, benign prostatic hypertrophy (BPH), tumor, or **an occluded Foley catheter**, and it can often be diagnosed by placing (or replacing) a Foley in the bladder. If urine output does not improve with the catheter in place, a renal ultrasound may be performed; hydronephrosis (dilation of the renal pelvis) may be present if the process is postrenal.

Laboratory findings aid in distinguishing prerenal from intrinsic renal failure. In prerenal failure, the kidney is not damaged and avidly reabsorbs sodium in order to hold on to water. As a result, urinary sodium is lower in prerenal (usually < 20 mEq/L) than in intrinsic renal failure (usually > 40 mEq/L). Similarly, the fractional excretion of sodium, or FENa, is typically < 1 in prerenal, and > 1 in postrenal failure (remember: FENa = 100 x (U/P sodium)/(U/P creatinine). Because the undamaged kidney also reabsorbs urea, the serum BUN:creatinine ratio is usually > 20:1 in prerenal failure, and < 20:1 in intrinsic renal failure.

Thromboembolic disease of the renal arteries can cause intrinsic renal failure. Thrombosis, the formation of a blood clot (thrombus), may result from atherosclerosis of the renal vessels or from emboli originating in other vessels or the heart. Acute renal failure is more likely to result from embolization to both renal arteries, which also generally causes flank pain, hematuria, and hypertension. Acute renal vein thrombosis can also cause acute renal failure, and usually occurs in children and young adults. It is associated with nephrotic syndrome, pregnancy, oral contraceptives, and dehydrated infants. In the elderly, renal vein thrombosis is usually gradual, and presents with hypertension and recurrent pulmonary emboli. Renal artery stenosis accounts for 2-5% of cases of hypertension and is usually due to atherosclerosis of the renal arteries.

Severe hemolytic transfusion reactions, which are usually due to ABO blood group incompatibility, typically occur immediately after transfusion. They can cause fever, chills, hypotension, disseminated intravascular coagulation (DIC), and acute renal failure due to massive amounts of hemoglobin causing tubular necrosis. Hemolytic transfusion reactions due to incompatibility of minor antigens (e.g., Duffy antigen) may be delayed by several days, and are usually less severe.

Fauci, 14th ed., pp 1558-59.
Tierney, 38th ed., pp 867-69.

9

(Block 1: Item 9)

(C)

Multiple myeloma is a plasma cell malignancy characterized by replacement of the bone marrow by monoclonal plasma cells; the malignant plasma cells typically overproduce monoclonal immunoglobulins and/or monoclonal light chains (kappa or lambda). The average age of presentation is 60 years. Bone marrow replacement initially causes anemia, then leukopenia and thrombocytopenia. Bone pain, especially in the back or ribs, and pathologic fractures are common. Patients may also present with infection due to neutropenia and an impaired antibody response (hypogammaglobulinemia). Renal failure can occur as a result of hypercalcemia and amyloid deposits, hyperuricemia, and high levels of immunoglobulin light chains filtered by the kidney. Patients are typically pale and have bone tenderness. There are several characteristic laboratory findings. Anemia is virtually always found (but, not in Stage I disease), often with rouleaux formation seen on the peripheral smear (the morphology of several red blood cells piled up on each other). Most patients will have a monoclonal spike on serum protein electrophoresis (SPEP), reflecting increased amounts of antibody produced by the single malignant clone of plasma cells. Hypercalcemia (secondary to lytic lesions caused by tumor expansion and the activation of osteoclasts by myeloma cells' secretion of activation factors) and an elevated creatinine (reflecting renal failure) are usually present. Uric acid is also elevated (note that renal failure and thiazide diuretics can further elevate uric acid). Alkaline phosphatase is not elevated despite bony involvement. Bone marrow biopsy shows variable amounts of plasma cell infiltration. X-rays may show lytic lesions in the skull, spine, proximal long bones, and ribs. Treatment includes systemic chemotherapy and control of pain, hypercalcemia, anemia, renal failure, and infections. Hypercalcemia responds well to glucocorticoids, hydration, natriuresis, calcitonin, and bisphosphonates.

Pancreatic carcinoma generally causes vague abdominal pain; pain radiating to the back often predominates. Obstruction of the biliary system often causes jaundice. There may be a mild anemia, hyperglycemia, and elevated liver function tests (reflecting obstructive jaundice). CT, MRI, and ERCP (endoscopic retrograde cholangiopancreatography) are usually the most helpful diagnostic tools. Several conditions including malignancy (paraneoplastic syndromes), hyperparathyroidism, vitamin D intoxication, milk-alkali syndrome, and thiazide diuretics can cause hypercalcemia. Hypercalcemia can cause constipation, polyuria, altered mental status, renal failure, and ventricular arrhythmias. Thiazides can cause **hypercalcemia** by increasing calcium reabsorption by the kidney. This is in contrast to loop diuretics, which lead to calcium loss by the kidney. **Primary hyperparathyroidism** is caused by hypersecretion of parathyroid hormone (PTH), usually by a parathyroid adenoma, and occasionally by parathyroid hyperplasia or carcinoma. PTH mobilizes calcium from bone, increases renal calcium reabsorption, and increases intestinal calcium absorption by increasing vitamin D formation. Excessive bone resorption induced by PTH can result in diffuse demineralization, pathologic fractures, and cystic bone lesions. Calcium-containing kidney stones commonly form in the urinary tract. (Remember that hyperparathyroidism involves "bones, stones, abdominal groans, and psychic moans.") Although serum calcium is high, serum phosphate is typically low (< 2.5 mg/dL) since PTH decreases renal phosphate reabsorption. Elevated serum PTH levels confirm the diagnosis. **Renal cell carcinoma** presents with hematuria, and sometimes with flank pain or abdominal mass. Anemia is common, and hypercalcemia occurs in approximately 10% of cases.

Fauci, 14th ed., pp 714-16.
Nicoll, 2nd ed., pp 181.
Tierney, 38th ed., pp 518-19, 676, 849, 927, 1085-86.

10

(Block 1: Item 10)

(C)

The etiologies of thrombocytopenia (platelet count < 150,000/μl) can be divided into three categories: (1) increased platelet destruction or platelet sequestration—hypersplenism, thrombotic thrombocytopenic purpura (TTP), hemolytic uremic syndrome, disseminated intravascular coagulation (DIC), and immunologic thrombocytopenia; (2) decreased platelet production—bone marrow replacement by malignancy or fibrosis, viral infections, and marrow suppressing drugs like alcohol; and (3) ineffective platelet production—folate or vitamin B_{12} deficiency.

Immunologic thrombocytopenia occurs when platelets are coated with antibody, immune complexes, or complement, and are consequently destroyed by mononuclear cells in the spleen and elsewhere. The principal causes are drugs, infections, and an autoimmune disorder referred to as idiopathic thrombocytopenic purpura (ITP). Many drugs (e.g., thiazides, several antibiotics) can cause thrombocytopenia and most cause platelet destruction by drug-antibody complexes that activate complement. **Heparin causes thrombocytopenia** in 5-15% of patients receiving therapeutic doses, and can cause severe bleeding, platelet aggregation, and paradoxical thrombosis. This usually occurs a few days after the start of heparin therapy, and is mostly due to drug-antibody complexes binding to platelets, and possibly also due to direct platelet agglutination by heparin. A patient with pre-existing mesenteric venous thrombosis would likely be 'exposed' to therapeutic doses of heparin for several days. Platelet counts often drop below 50,000/μl, the prothrombin time (PT) is normal, and the partial thromboplastin time (PTT) is elevated (secondary to heparin therapy). Immediate cessation of heparin will reverse the thrombocytopenia and the heparin-induced thrombosis.

ITP (immune or idiopathic thrombocytopenic purpura) is characterized by a low platelet count in the absence of other causes of thrombocytopenia. It is an autoimmune process that occurs primarily in children and young women. Children usually present with sudden onset of bruising and petechiae, while adults present with chronic bruising or incidental thrombocytopenia. ITP is occasionally associated with a mild anemia, and coagulation studies (PT and PTT) are normal. **TTP** is characterized by thrombocytopenia and microangiopathic hemolytic anemia. In contrast to ITP, it occurs primarily in adults and platelets are consumed by clotting reactions as a result of the microangiopathic changes, not by autoimmune destruction. TTP may also cause neurological symptoms and renal failure. Laboratory findings include severe anemia with fragmented red blood cells (schistocytes) and elevated BUN and creatinine. Coagulation studies (PT and PTT) are generally normal. Hemolytic uremic syndrome (HUS) is similar to TTP; in children it often occurs after infection with certain bacteria such as *E. coli* stain O157:H7. **DIC** occurs in association with serious underlying illness such as sepsis, and is characterized by general activation of the clotting system, leading to both bleeding and thrombosis. DIC results in thrombocytopenia, prolonged PT and

PTT, increased D-dimer (a fibrin degradation product), and decreased fibrinogen. **Acute adrenal insufficiency** (adrenal crisis) is caused by inadequate corticosteroid secretion by the adrenal gland. It commonly occurs in primary adrenocortical insufficiency (Addison's disease) which is usually an autoimmune disease, and can occur following a major stress such as trauma or surgery. Findings include weakness, hypotension, hyperkalemia, hyponatremia, hypoglycemia, mild anemia, eosinophilia, and decreased 24-hour urine cortisol.

Fauci, 14th ed., pp 731-32.
Ferri, 3rd ed., pp 374-75, 495-98.
Tierney, 38th ed., pp 520-24, 531-33, 1094.

11

(Block 1: Item 11)

(B)

Ethanol is a sedative-hypnotic whose toxicity is dose-dependent, although tolerance varies widely. Ataxia generally occurs with blood levels over 100 mg/dL, and patients with blood levels over 200 mg/dL become drowsy and confused (in California, driving with a level above 80 mg/dL is illegal). Respiratory depression and death can occur at levels over 400 mg/dL. Since chronic alcoholism causes thiamine deficiency, prompt administration of thiamine to comatose patients can improve or prevent Wernicke's encephalopathy (see answer 16). Ethanol acutely causes peripheral vasodilation, causing a mild drop in blood pressure, a compensatory mild tachycardia, and increase in cardiac output. **Benzodiazepines** are also sedative-hypnotics, and they depress mental and respiratory function. They have additive effects on CNS depression when combined with other drugs of this class such as ethanol. Benzodiazepine toxicity can be reversed with flumazenil, a benzodiazepine antagonist.

In contrast to the sedative-hypnotics, **cocaine** causes CNS and sympathetic stimulation, although CNS depression can develop subsequently as a rebound effect. Effects of cocaine include hyperactivity, euphoria, hypertension, and tachycardia. Death can occur as a result of seizure, stroke, myocardial infarction, or CNS depression. A cocaine metabolite, benzoylecgonine, is usually detected in the urine of abusers for 24-96 hours after use (even longer for chronic, heavy abusers). Phencyclidine **(PCP)** is a dissociative anesthetic that can cause agitation, hypertension, tachycardia, and nystagmus. Stupor can progress to coma, respiratory failure, and death. **Salicylate** toxicity, as occurs with aspirin overdose, can cause nausea, vomiting, tinnitus, and fever. Severe intoxications can lead to lethargy, convulsions, coma, and respiratory failure. Salicylates initially cause hyperventilation and a respiratory alkalosis, followed by a metabolic acidosis. Salicylates are readily detectable in the blood.

Carey, 29th ed., pp 513, 519-22.
Fauci, 14th ed., p 2205.

12

(Block 1: Item 12)

(B)

Foreign body aspiration results in significant morbidity and mortality in childhood, particularly between the ages of 6 months and 4 years. Deaths are primarily due to upper airway obstruction, which can present with acute cyanosis, choking, cough, stridor, or inability to vocalize. A foreign body lodged in the esophagus can also impair respiration by compressing the airway. Foreign body aspiration into the lower respiratory tract can be more difficult to diagnose, because it may not cause immediate symptoms. The diagnosis should be considered in any child with acute onset of cough, choking, or wheezing, as well as chronic cough or wheezing, or recurrent pneumonia. Suspicion is higher still for children with access to peanuts, hard candy or other items that are easily aspirated. When a foreign body is lodged in the lower respiratory tract, symptoms of cough and wheezing may initially improve, but can recur after a latent period of minutes to months. When bronchus (or bronchiole) obstruction allows air entry but not exit, then hyperinflation occurs. If air cannot move in or out, then atelectasis ensues distal to the obstruction. In either case, the foreign body can induce non-specific inflammation, and if long-standing, can cause bronchiectasis (dilation of bronchi or bronchioles), lung abscess, and empyema (purulent pleural fluid). Abscesses typically contain anaerobes from the oral cavity that are aspirated along with the foreign body, such as *Bacteroides*, *Fusobacterium* and *Peptostreptococcus*. On physical exam, a foreign body can cause localized wheezing or asymmetric breath sounds. On chest X-ray, inspiratory films may show localized hyperinflation due to air-trapping, while forced expiratory films may accentuate the local hyperinflation and mediastinal shift to the opposite side, since the obstruction prevents emptying of the affected side, while the unaffected side is able to empty. This child's chest X-ray (right middle lobe infiltrate with large pleural effusion) underscores the propensity for foreign objects to preferentially lodge in the right side of the pulmonary tree due to the gentler slope of the right mainstem bronchus. Definitive diagnosis may require direct visualization by bronchoscopy.

Cystic fibrosis (CF), the most common fatal genetic disease in the U.S., is the major cause of severe chronic lung disease in children (though some cases are not diagnosed until adulthood). It is also associated with pancreatic insufficiency, sinusitis, nasal polyposis, and rectal prolapse. CF often presents with failure to thrive or recurrent respiratory infections, and the diagnosis is made with a positive sweat test or genotyping. Pulmonary findings include productive cough and wheezing. Bronchiectasis can cause hemoptysis, and airways are typically colonized with *Pseudomonas aeruginosa*.
Immunodeficiencies often cause recurrent or severe infections. Examples include IgA deficiency, X-linked (Bruton's) hypogammaglobulinemia, thymic aplasia (DiGeorge's syndrome), severe combined immunodeficiency (SCID), and deficiency of complement factors. IgA deficiency causes recurrent sinus and lung infections. X-linked (Bruton's) hypogammaglobulinemia results in recurrent pyogenic infections, especially in the

respiratory tract. Thymic aplasia (DiGeorge's syndrome) causes severe viral, fungal, and protozoal infections. Severe combined immunodeficiency (SCID), where both B and T cell function is impaired, is associated with bacterial, viral, fungal, and protozoal infections. Patients with deficiency of complement factors C6, C7, or C8 are particularly susceptible to *Neisseria* infections. **Ingestion of hydrocarbons** such as benzene, gasoline, or kerosene can cause vomiting, respiratory distress, fever, and central nervous system depression. Aspiration, suggested by a history of coughing, can result in hydrocarbon pneumonitis (edema, inflammation, and hemorrhage). Chest X-ray shows extensive diffuse infiltrates. **Appendicitis** typically causes low-grade fever and periumbilical pain that migrates to the right lower quadrant. It may also cause anorexia, vomiting, diarrhea, and constipation. Pneumonia or urinary tract infection may occasionally be confused for subacute appendicitis in children.

Behrman, 15th ed., pp 734-37, 1205-08, 1215-16.
Hay, 13th ed., pp 439-41, 447-48, 547-48, 804-11.

13

(Block 1: Item 13)

(B)

Guillain-Barré syndrome (GBS), also known as acute idiopathic polyneuropathy, is an acute inflammatory demyelinating polyradiculopathy (affects nerve roots) that primarily causes motor deficits. It is the most common cause of acute paralytic illness, and typically occurs in young adults. Approximately two thirds of patients have a respiratory or gastrointestinal illness, such as *Campylobacter jejuni* gastroenteritis, within 30 days prior to the onset of neurological symptoms. There is thought to be an immunological basis for this syndrome, but its mechanism is unclear. The principal manifestation is symmetric weakness, which typically begins in the lower extremities and may spread upward to involve the arms and one or both sides of the face (ascending paralysis). Swallowing (due to cranial nerve involvement) and respiration (due to intercostal muscle weakness) may also be impaired. Reflexes are depressed or absent bilaterally. Sensory manifestations are much less prominent, but can include "glove and stocking" anesthesia and radicular pain. Autonomic dysfunction can cause tachycardia or bradycardia, hypertension or hypotension, and loss of sphincter control. The cerebrospinal fluid (CSF) in GBS typically shows elevated protein (mostly IgG) and normal to slightly elevated lymphocytes. However, these CSF changes can take 2 or 3 weeks to develop. Electrophysiologic studies reveal slowed conduction velocities. Patients with GBS need close respiratory monitoring, and may require mechanical ventilation. Respiratory failure is the main cause of mortality in GBS. Intravenous immunoglobulin has been found to be helpful and is usually the first-line treatment. Plasmapheresis (plasma exchange) is also helpful, but is generally reserved for severe cases with respiratory impairment, since it imposes significant stress on the cardiovascular system. The use of intravenous steroids is controversial, but appears to adversely affect outcome. Mortality from GBS is approximately 3%. Recovery can take several months, and 10-20% of patients have residual motor deficits.

Acute disseminated encephalomyelitis (ADEM) is a demyelinating disease of the brain and spinal cord that is frequently associated with recent immunization or infection. It may be confused with acute multiple sclerosis. ADEM has occurred after the administration of smallpox vaccines and certain rabies vaccines. It occurs most commonly after childhood viral exanthems, such as measles and varicella (chickenpox). As with GBS, an immunological mechanism is postulated but not proven. Signs and symptoms of ADEM include fever, headache, meningismus, lethargy, seizures, quadriparesis or hemiparesis, and extensor plantar responses (upgoing toes representing upper motor neuron lesions). MRI shows extensive white matter involvement in the brain and spinal cord. In **myasthenia gravis** (MG), antibodies against the post-synaptic acetylcholine receptor block neuromuscular transmission, resulting in muscle weakness. It is associated with thymomas, thyroid disease, rheumatoid arthritis, and systemic lupus erythematosus (SLE). MG classically causes diplopia and ptosis. Muscles of respiration and of the extremities may also be involved. Weakness worsens with exercise and improves with rest. Neither sensation nor reflexes are affected. The diagnosis of MG is confirmed by the improvement of muscle strength in response to an anticholinesterase such as edrophonium (Tensilon). **Poliomyelitis**, which is caused by the fecal-orally-transmitted poliovirus and causes degeneration of the anterior horn cells of the spinal cord, has become rare in the developed world due to an effective vaccine. Most cases in the U.S. are now vaccine-associated (there is a small risk of developing disease with the OPV vaccine). When infection does occur, it is usually asymptomatic, or it results in "abortive poliomyelitis," with fever, headache, vomiting, and diarrhea. It can also cause "non-paralytic poliomyelitis," which causes the above symptoms as well as signs of aseptic meningitis, or "paralytic poliomyelitis," which includes muscle paralysis, tremors, and constipation. Weakness or paralysis may occur in muscles supplied by spinal nerves (affecting limbs and respiration) as well as cranial nerves (affecting swallowing and facial muscles). Poliomyelitis can resemble GBS, but the weakness in GBS is usually more ascending and symmetric. **Polymyositis** is a systemic disease of unknown etiology. Its main manifestation is bilateral weakness of proximal muscles, especially of the limbs. The disease is called dermatomyositis when it is associated with characteristic skin manifestations, such as purplish flushing of the eyelids, periorbital edema, and a red rash of the face, neck, shoulders, and torso ("heliotrope rash"). Dermatomyositis can be associated with occult malignancy, such as ovarian cancer.

Fauci, 14th ed., pp 2418-19.
Ferri, 3rd ed., pp 705-08, 1268-69.
Tierney, 38th ed., pp 817, 978, 985-86.

14

(Block 1: Item 14)

(D)

Mitral stenosis is frequently the result of rheumatic heart disease (RHD), which produces rigidity and deformity of valve leaflets and fusion of commissures and chordae tendineae. (Recall that the frequency of valves affected by rheumatic heart disease is mitral > aortic > tricuspid > pulmonic.) Mitral stenosis may also be due to progressive scarring or calcification, congenital defects, or rare causes such as endomyocardial fibroelastosis, carcinoid syndrome, or systemic lupus erythematosus (SLE). A narrowed mitral valve area produces a heart murmur, which is mid-diastolic, low pitched (a rumble), and located at the apex. [Remember that when you "**AS**k **MI**," I'll tell you which valve lesions cause systolic murmurs (AS = aortic stenosis, MI = mitral insufficiency). That leaves aortic insufficiency and mitral stenosis, which cause diastolic murmurs.] With sufficient valve area narrowing, left atrial pressure must increase to maintain flow across the valve. Dyspnea and fatigue worsen when left atrial pressures rise enough to produce pulmonary venous congestion. Pulmonary venous hypertension is seen on chest X-ray in the form of pulmonary vasculature redistribution to the upper lung fields. Pulmonary venous hypertension induces anastomoses between pulmonary and bronchial veins which often rupture and cause hemoptysis. Most patients with mitral stenosis develop atrial fibrillation, which further exacerbates dyspnea and fatigue. In addition to the mid-diastolic murmur, an opening snap is heard in early diastole as a result of valve thickening. Electrocardiogram (ECG) shows broad notched P-waves, which represent left atrial enlargement, and often atrial fibrillation.

The best way to evaluate mitral stenosis is **echocardiography**. Echocardiography demonstrates thickened valves that open and close poorly. The valve area can be measured, and the pressure gradient as well as the pulmonary artery pressure can be estimated with Doppler techniques. Echocardiography can demonstrate if the left atrium is enlarged, which increases the likelihood of atrial fibrillation and systemic embolization, thus necessitating anticoagulation. It may also reveal an atrial myxoma, which can present like mitral stenosis. Correction of the stenosis with mitral commissurotomy, balloon valvuloplasty, or replacement with a prosthetic valve may be done depending on symptoms and the extent of valve damage.

In the rare case where echocardiography cannot sufficiently determine the severity of obstruction, **coronary catheterization and angiography** is used to decide whether correction of the stenosis is indicated. It also helps to assess associated lesions such as aortic stenosis or insufficiency. Coronary catheterization is also recommended in men over 45, women over 55, and in those with coronary risk factors, in order to detect coronary artery stenoses that can be bypassed at the time of surgery. In the evaluation of blood-tinged sputum, **bronchoscopy** should be performed if there is reason to suspect lung cancer, i.e. if the patient is a smoker, over age 40, and has had symptoms for more than one week. Blood-tinged sputum in an otherwise healthy nonsmoker is usually secondary to acute bronchitis, and extensive evaluation is usually not immediately necessary. **Pulmonary angiography** is the definitive test for diagnosis of pulmonary embolism. It is most useful when the clinical suspicion of pulmonary embolism differs significantly from the results of a ventilation/perfusion (V/Q) scan and when the V/Q scan is of intermediate probability. **Pulmonary catheterization** involves inserting a catheter (Swan-Ganz catheter) into a suitable vein (e.g., femoral, subclavian, internal jugular) and floating it into the superior vena cava, right atrium, right ventricle, pulmonary artery, and pulmonary wedge positions. It allows measurement of right atrial, right ventricular, pulmonary artery, and pulmonary capillary wedge (which estimates left atrial) pressures, oxygen saturation, cardiac output, and other hemodynamic measurements. This can be critical in the evaluation of cardiogenic shock, septic shock, myocardial infarction, and other entities. Of course, this is much more invasive than echocardiography, which can also be used to evaluate some of these disorders.

Fauci, 14th ed., pp 1311-15, 1470.
Ferri, 3rd ed., pp 229-31.
Novelline, 5th ed., pp 188-89.
Tierney, 38th ed., pp 257, 344-45, 349-53, 419.

15

(Block 1: Item 15)

(D)

Tetralogy of Fallot is the third most common cyanotic congenital cardiac lesion in the neonatal period. There are four characteristic abnormalities: (1) an overriding, large ascending aorta, (2) right ventricular outflow tract obstruction [infundibular stenosis, pulmonary valve stenosis, or a combination of the two], (3) a large ventricular septal defect (VSD), and (4) right ventricular hypertrophy secondary to pulmonary artery stenosis. In tetralogy of Fallot, up to 75% of deoxygenated venous blood returning to the heart may pass into the aorta without becoming oxygenated; this is due to right-to-left shunting across the VSD and decreased pulmonary flow. Neonates with tetralogy commonly present with varying degrees of cyanosis; they may also have "tet spells" with periodic cyanosis, diaphoresis and agitation (caused by an increase in the right ventricular outflow resistance and a concomitant increase in the right-to-left shunt). On cardiac exam, "tet" infants will have a loud systolic ejection murmur (heard best in the left upper sternal border) due to right ventricular outflow obstruction. ECG demonstrates right atrial dilatation and right ventricular hypertrophy. Chest X-ray may show a small boot-shaped heart and decreased pulmonary vascular markings. Prior to surgical correction or palliation, cardiac catheterization is essential; the success of operative treatment depends on the size of the pulmonary arteries. Fortunately, surgical correction of the defects has been quite successful in reversing these dynamics.

Other cyanotic congenital cardiac lesions include **T**runcus arteriosis, **T**otal anomalous pulmonary venous return, **T**ransposition of the great arteries, and **T**ricuspid atresia (other rare, cyanotic "zebras" exist). **Total anomalous pulmonary venous return** (TAPVR) is a rare cardiac lesion where the pulmonary veins drain back into the right atrium, either directly or indirectly through other venous channels (brachiocephalic vein, SVC, coronary sinus, portal or hepatic veins). All systemic and pulmonary venous blood returns to the right atrium, which can either cross the tricuspid valve to the right ventricle or shunt to the left atrium across an ASD to the left ventricle. Pulmonary vascular resistance, obstruction to pulmonary venous drainage, and the presence of arterial and venous level shunts are key factors in the hemodynamics. Depending on the presence and degree of right-to-left shunting at the atrial level, left ventricular output is either maintained or decreased; right ventricular output is greatly increased resulting in pulmonary venous hypertension, pulmonary edema, and pulmonary arterial hypertension. Patients with TAPVR often have severe cyanosis, a small heart (poor cardiac function) and edematous lungs (dyspnea). **Atrial septal defects** account for 8% of congenital heart lesions and do not cause cyanosis until very advanced stages of disease, where pulmonary hypertension occurs. There are four different types of lesions (ostium secundum, ostium primum, sinus venosis, and coronary sinus defects). Unlike tetralogy, ASD favors a left-to-right shunt at the atrial level, thus increasing flow across the tricuspid and pulmonary valves and increasing pulmonary blood flow. Although ASDs are not routinely associated with symptoms, children may have slow weight gain and repeated pulmonary infections. **Endocardial fibroelastosis** is a rare form of focal or diffuse, fibroelastic thickening of the endocardium, typically not producing cyanosis. The cartilage-like thickening most often affects the mural left ventricular endocardium and is often associated with another type of cardiac anomaly (33% of cases have aortic valve obstruction). Depending on the extent of the fibroelastic disease, it can either have no clinical significance or progress to rapid, debilitating cardiac decompensation in children (usually under 2 years old). **Anomalies of the coronary vessels** can include anomalous origin from the aorta, anomalous origin from the pulmonary artery, fistulous connections of the coronary vessels, and anomalies of the coronary sinus. The most frequent morphological anomaly of the coronary sinus is persistence of a left superior vena cava, which drains through the orifice of the coronary sinus. The "unroofed" coronary sinus syndrome with persistent left superior vena cava (SVC) occurs when part or the entire common wall between the coronary sinus and the left atrium is absent, so that deoxygenated blood reaches the left atrium. This rare lesion produces cyanosis, and also risks cerebral embolization and abscess.

Cotran, 5th ed., pp 561-62.
Marino, 1st ed., pp 16-19.
Way, 10th ed., pp 400-01.
http://www.pediheart.org/practitioners/defects

16

(Block 1: Item 16)

(C)

Chronic alcohol abuse can cause liver disease, anemia, cardiomyopathy, pancreatitis, and a myriad of central nervous system (CNS) disorders. CNS effects due to alcohol toxicity or secondary nutritional deficiencies include: restless sleep, peripheral neuropathy, cerebellar degeneration (unsteady gait often with nystagmus), impaired cognition and memory (which may become permanent), anxiety, hallucinations, Wernicke's syndrome, and Korsakoff's syndrome. Wernicke's syndrome, also known as Wernicke's encephalopathy, is caused by thiamine (vitamin B_1) deficiency and classically consists of the triad of confusion, ataxia, and ophthalmoplegia (usually due to sixth nerve palsy). **Parenteral (IV or IM) thiamine administration** early in its course generally results in dramatic improvement, although approximately half of patients are left with permanent gait instability. *Glucose infusions may precipitate or worsen Wernicke's encephalopathy. For this reason, thiamine should be given prior to glucose (or dextrose) administration.* Another sequela of Wernicke's encephalopathy is Korsakoff's syndrome, also known as Korsakoff's psychosis, which is characterized by amnesia and confabulation (making up stories about past events, usually to disguise an inability to remember them). When Korsakoff's psychosis occurs together with other components of Wernicke's encephalopathy, it is termed Wernicke-Korsakoff syndrome. Like Wernicke's encephalopathy, Korsakoff's psychosis results from thiamine deficiency in alcoholics with poor nutrition. Patients with malnutrition from other causes, such as starvation, cancer, and AIDS, are also at risk. Thiamine is a cofactor for several enzymes, and its deficiency causes a decrease in cerebral glucose utilization that results in mitochondrial damage.

Alcohol withdrawal occurs when someone stops drinking after a prolonged period of alcohol consumption. Four withdrawal states are described, though they can overlap: the "shakes," withdrawal seizures, hallucinosis, and delirium tremens (DTs). The "shakes" or "jitters" occur 12-48 hours after reduction of intake (the day after admission to the hospital, for example) and are associated with agitation and tachycardia. They can be treated with **diazepam** (Valium), chlordiazepoxide (Librium), or if the patient has significant liver disease, lorazepam (Ativan). **Fluid and electrolytes** need to be carefully monitored and replaced when needed. Patients in alcohol withdrawal may be dehydrated due to vomiting, sweating, or fever. In addition, they often have **hypomagnesemia**, hypokalemia, and hypophosphatemia. Withdrawal seizures usually occur from 7 to 30 hours after drinking ceases. The seizures are generalized, often recur within 6 hours, and can be treated with lorazepam (Ativan) or diazepam (Valium). Hallucinations associated with alcohol withdrawal, like any psychosis, can be treated with antipsychotics such as haloperidol (Haldol). DTs usually occur within one week of reduction of alcohol intake, and are characterized by shakiness, confusion, tachycardia, hypertension, sweating, nausea, vomiting, and fever. This is the most dangerous form of alcohol withdrawal with a mortality rate of approximately 15%. Treatment includes monitoring, supportive therapy, and sedation in an intensive care unit.

Chronic alcoholics often have coagulopathies because hepatocyte loss leads to depletion of coagulation factors, especially II, VII, IX, X and Protein C and S (the liver synthesizes all coagulation factors except factor VIII). Depletion of these factors is exacerbated by nutritional vitamin K deficiency, since vitamin K is a cofactor in the production of these factors. Alcoholics often have a prolonged serum prothrombin time; hence, **administration of an anticoagulant** would only potentiate the coagulopathy. Alcohol can also cause thrombocytopenia by its bone marrow depressant effects. **Vitamin C** is used to treat scurvy, in which vitamin C deficiency results in defective collagen formation and poor blood vessel integrity. As a result, patients have a tendency to bleed, and present with perifollicular hemorrhages, petechiae and purpura, and bleeding gums.

Fauci, 14th ed., pp 1704-05, 2455, 2504.
Ferri, 3rd ed., pp 172-77.
Tierney, 38th ed., pp 530, 968, 1035, 1192.

17

(Block 1: Item 17)

(E)

A patient with fever, malaise, a red sore throat (with or without exudates) and tender cervical lymphadenopathy may have streptococcal pharyngitis or pharyngitis caused by Epstein-Barr virus (EBV; causes infectious mononucleosis), adenovirus, or other infectious agents. Suspicion of mononucleosis should rise if symptoms do not resolve after 3 to 5 days, which is typical of streptococcal pharyngitis. Mononucleosis can occur at any age, but typically occurs between the ages of 10 and 35. It is likely transmitted by saliva (the "kissing disease") and has an incubation period of a few weeks. Symptoms include sore throat, fever, malaise, anorexia, and myalgias. Findings on physical exam include tender lymphadenopathy (classically in the posterior cervical chain), splenomegaly, and pharyngitis (can be accompanied by tonsillar enlargement and exudate similar to streptococcal pharyngitis). A maculopapular rash occurs in about 15% of cases. The rash occurs in almost everyone who is given ampicillin, but this is a very embarrassing method of diagnosing mononucleosis! Laboratory findings typically include an elevated lymphocyte count with numerous "atypical" large lymphocytes (which are T cells reacting to infected host cells). Mild anemia and thrombocytopenia may occur. Heterophil antibodies (and the related Monospot test) are usually present and quite specific for **EBV**. [There is a long list of etiologies for "heterophile-negative mononucleosis," including cytomegalovirus (CMV), heterophile-negative EBV, hepatitis viruses, and HIV.] If heterophile antibodies are negative, and there is high suspicion for EBV, the test may be repeated in 1-2 weeks, or blood can be tested for antibodies to EBV. Positive anti-VCA (viral capsid antibodies) IgM is the most helpful serologic finding when the heterophile test is negative. Anti-VCA IgG and antibodies to EBV nuclear antigen (EBNA) remain positive for life and are therefore less useful in distinguishing recent infection from previous infection. Hepatic aminotransferases (AST and ALT) are commonly elevated, as infectious mononucleosis can also cause hepatitis. No specific treatment for infectious mononucleosis is available, and symptoms usually resolve in a few weeks, though they may persist for months.

Rheumatic fever is a systemic immune-mediated illness that occurs after group A streptococcal (*Streptococcus pyogenes*) pharyngitis. Recall that group A streptococcal skin infections are not associated with rheumatic fever, but are more likely to cause immune-complex (post-streptococcal) glomerulonephritis. Rheumatic fever typically occurs in children, 1-4 weeks after the pharyngitis. Diagnosis is based on the Jones criteria: carditis, polyarthritis, erythema marginatum and subcutaneous nodules, and Sydenham's chorea. Carditis can include pericarditis, cardiomegaly, congestive heart failure, or mitral or aortic regurgitation. Erythema marginatum is a rash consisting of macules with clear centers, and subcutaneous nodules are uncommon except in children. The arthritis in rheumatic fever is a migratory polyarthritis that sequentially involves the large joints. Sydenham's chorea (involuntary movements of the face, tongue, and upper extremities) is the least common but most diagnostic sign of rheumatic fever. Laboratory data that supports the diagnosis of rheumatic fever includes evidence of a recent group A streptococcal pharyngitis (throat culture or rapid antigen test), and high or increasing titers of the antistreptococcal antibodies, **antistreptolysin O (ASO)** or anti-DNase B. Although treatment of streptococcal pharyngitis with penicillin does not generally alleviate symptoms, it is critical for prevention of rheumatic fever (and less commonly, glomerulonephritis). Recurrence of rheumatic fever can be prevented with prophylactic penicillin. Rheumatic fever usually results in rheumatic heart disease, which affects the heart valves (mitral > aortic > tricuspid > pulmonic). Note that up to 20% of individuals in certain populations are asymptomatic carriers of group A strep. There are no definitive guidelines for the management of those whose cultures remain positive after treatment.

Antiplatelet antibodies are positive in some autoimmune thrombocytopenias, such as idiopathic thrombocytopenia (ITP), which occurs primarily in children and young women. Children usually present with sudden onset of bruising and petechiae, while adults present with chronic bruising or are diagnosed when platelets are incidentally found to be low. There is usually no systemic illness and the spleen is not palpable. **Bone marrow aspiration or biopsy** may be considered in the evaluation of pancytopenia, anemia, suspected leukemia or myelodysplastic syndromes, lymphoma and fever of unknown origin (FUO). Viral **hepatitis** typically begins with a prodrome of anorexia, nausea, vomiting, malaise, and symptoms of upper respiratory infection. Although viral hepatitis can cause heterophile-negative mononucleosis, most patients are jaundiced, have an enlarged and tender liver, and have markedly elevated AST and ALT (in the 100s to 1000s range).

Fauci, 14th ed., pp 337, 677, 784, 886-87.
Nicoll, 2nd ed., pp 81, 109, 147.
Tierney, 38th ed., pp 417-19, 640-44, 1291-92.

18

(Block 1: Item 18)

(A)

Acute aortic dissection is an entity in the differential diagnosis of chest pain that must not be missed, because it is lethal if left untreated. It occurs most commonly in hypertensive men between the ages of 60 and 80. The dissection begins at the site of a tear in the vessel's intima, and generally proceeds distally. Aortic dissections involving the ascending aorta or the aortic arch are classified as Type A (proximal) dissections. Those limited to the descending aorta are classified as Type B (distal) dissections. Patients with structural abnormalities of the aorta, such as Marfan's syndrome, more commonly suffer proximal dissections. Pregnancy, bicuspid aortic valve, and coarctation of the aorta predispose to both proximal and distal dissection. Hypertension contributes to the propagation of dissection, which may extend to the abdominal aorta. Dissection can also extend proximally to the aortic root. Death is usually due to aortic rupture (which can cause cardiac tamponade) or acute aortic regurgitation with left ventricular failure. Symptoms of aortic dissection include acute onset of severe chest pain that is described as sharp, tearing, or ripping. Its location may be in the anterior chest in a proximal dissection, or it may radiate to the back in a distal dissection. It may progress to the abdomen as the dissection proceeds down the abdominal aorta. The pain occasionally radiates to the arms and neck. Occlusion of the carotid or vertebral arteries may cause syncope or hemiplegia. Classic signs of aortic dissection include unequal peripheral pulses and blood pressures and a diastolic murmur of aortic insufficiency due to dissection near the aortic valve. Chest X-ray classically reveals a widened superior mediastinum with an abnormal aortic contour. The diagnosis can be made with CT, MRI, or angiography. Transesophageal echocardiography (TEE) or even transthoracic echocardiography (TTE) is also useful, and they can be performed quickly and at the bedside. Treatment includes blood pressure control, emergent surgical repair for all Type A dissections, and surgical repair of some Type B dissections.

Aortic dissection is most commonly confused with **acute myocardial infarction** (MI). Pain with a MI is often severe, and is described as crushing, pressing, burning, or aching. It is often a more severe form of angina pain that has recently been increasing in frequency as well as severity. The pain is typically retrosternal, and can radiate to the jaw, neck, left shoulder and arm. Other common symptoms are dyspnea and a cold sweat. Patients are anxious, diaphoretic, hypertensive (or hypotensive in patients with shock), and the heart exam may reveal a gallop (S_4 and/or S_3) and a systolic murmur of mitral regurgitation, which usually indicates papillary muscle dysfunction or even rupture. Electrocardiography (ECG) classically shows ST segment elevation or depression, evolving Q-waves, and symmetric T-wave inversions. Cardiac enzymes such as CK-MB and troponin I are elevated.

Pulmonary embolism (PE) is another important disease in the differential diagnosis of chest pain. The source of the embolism is usually a deep vein thrombosis

(DVT), and the diagnosis should be suspected when a patient has been immobilized, or is otherwise hypercoagulable (e.g., recent surgery, malignancy), and develops chest pain, dyspnea, tachypnea, or tachycardia. Chest pain associated with PE is usually pleuritic, i.e. it changes with breathing and position. Chest X-ray is usually normal, but occasionally shows a wedge-shaped density with its apex directed toward the hilum, known as Hampton's hump, or an area of focal oligemia (fewer visible blood vessels due to lack of blood flow), known as Westermark's sign. ECG usually shows sinus tachycardia, but may reveal the classic S1Q3T3 pattern (wide S-wave in lead I, large Q-wave and inverted T-wave in lead III). Arterial blood gas shows hypoxemia. Pulmonary angiography is the definitive test for diagnosis of pulmonary embolism (but it is rarely performed). It is most useful when the clinical suspicion of pulmonary embolism differs significantly from the results of a ventilation/perfusion (V/Q) scan, and when the V/Q scan is of intermediate probability. Spiral chest CT-Angio (when available) can be used to confirm or rule out clinical suspicion of PE. **Spontaneous pneumothorax** (air in the pleural space) typically occurs in tall, thin men between the ages of 20 and 40. It may also occur secondary to various lung diseases, such as COPD, asthma, and cystic fibrosis. Symptoms include pleuritic chest pain on the affected side and dyspnea. Physical exam may reveal localized decreased breath sounds and hyperresonance, but the diagnosis is usually made on chest X-ray by visualization of the visceral pleura line, with no pulmonary vasculature markings beyond it. Acute arterial occlusion by an **embolus to the right subclavian artery** would cause sudden, excruciating extremity (right arm) pain. Major arterial occlusion causes the 5 **P's: p**ain, **p**allor, **p**ulselessness, tingling or numbness (**p**aresthesias), coolness (**p**oikilothermia), and **p**aralysis. If not corrected within a few hours by surgical embolectomy via cutdown and Fogarty balloon catheterization, limb loss will occur.

Blackbourne, 2nd ed., pp 453-54.
Friedman, 6th ed., pp 44-46.
Tierney, 38th ed., pp 300-01, 372-74, 456-57.

19

(Block 1: Item 19)

(A)

This patient is both hypercapnic (normal $PaCO_2$ is 35-45 mm Hg) and hypoxic (normal PaO_2 for a 50-year-old is ~83 mm Hg). Hypoxemia during emergence from anesthesia can be caused by hypoventilation, decreased functional residual capacity from anesthesia, weakness (from muscle relaxants), increased airway resistance, fluid overload, mucous plugging (with increased secretions), increased O_2 consumption (increased sympathetic drive), decreased FiO_2, or diffusion hypoxia. This is a long list! The patient's arterial hypercapnia and acidemia help narrow the differential. In acute respiratory acidosis, **alveolar hypoventilation** causes acute CO_2 retention. An increase in $PaCO_2$ of 10 mm Hg will cause a decrease in pH of about 0.08 and a compensatory increase in bicarbonate of about 1 mEq/L. (This is in contrast to chronic respiratory acidosis, where the same increase in $PaCO_2$ corresponds to a pH drop of only about 0.03 and a bicarbonate increase of about 3.5 mEq/L, since renal compensation has occurred.) Excessive CO_2 in alveoli displaces alveolar O_2 thus resulting in hypoxemia. The physiologic effects of hypercapnia occur not only as a result of increased arterial CO_2 but also through the resulting decrease in pH. Causes of acute respiratory acidosis include: central nervous system (CNS) depression by drugs such as anesthetics or by a cerebral event such as a stroke; acute airway obstruction as in foreign body aspiration or laryngospasm; severe pneumonia or pulmonary edema; impaired lung motion such as in hemothorax, pneumothorax, or flail chest; and ventilator dysfunction. Hypercapnia can cause ventricular arrhythmias and pulmonary vasoconstriction. Like hypoxemia, hypercapnia can result in increased myocardial O_2 demand (tachycardia, early hypertension) and decreased myocardial supply (tachycardia, late hypotension).

Occult hemorrhage can also cause hypotension, but it is unlikely to cause acute respiratory acidosis unless decreased CNS perfusion results in damage to the central respiratory center. Ventricular premature beats (VPCs or PVCs), also called ventricular extrasystoles, commonly occur in normal hearts and can be asymptomatic and benign. They may be caused by cardiac disease, electrolyte abnormalities, hyperthyroidism, or hypoxia. PVCs can progress to ventricular fibrillation. Especially in the postoperative patient, hypercapnia, hypoxemia, pain or fluid overload can precipitate PVCs. **Primary cardiac irritability and failure** is very unlikely in this scenario—PVCs are usually asymptomatic (benign) and, rarely, progress to cardiac failure. **Anesthetic gases** could cause diffusion hypoxia by directly displacing oxygen or by diluting alveolar CO_2; this would result in a decrease in respiratory drive and ventilation. Diffusion hypoxia is more common during emergence from anesthesia; a patient two hours postoperative would unlikely have high enough concentrations of anesthetic gases in their alveoli to cause diffusion hypoxia. A **pulmonary embolus** can cause a significant drop in PaO_2, but it also typically causes acute respiratory alkalosis due to hyperventilation (early on).

Ferri, 3rd ed., pp 186-94.
Tierney, 38th ed., pp 311-12, 395-96.
http://www.anesthesia.wisc.edu/Topics/Physiology/physiology.html

---

20

(Block 1: Item 20)

(C)

Polymyalgia rheumatica (PMR) is a clinical syndrome characterized by polymyalgias (pain) and polyarthralgias (stiffness) mainly of the back, shoulders, neck, and pelvic girdle muscles. These symptoms are typically worse in the morning (especially on awakening) and at night. PMR often coexists with temporal (giant cell) arteritis, which is a granulomatous inflammatory process, primarily of the arteries of the carotid system. Temporal arteritis classically presents with headache, tenderness and decreased pulsation over the temporal arteries, and scalp tenderness. Both disorders occur primarily in individuals over 50 years old. In addition to pain and stiffness, patients with PMR frequently have fever, malaise, and weight loss. Depression may also be present. Aside from tenderness of the aforementioned areas, physical examination is usually unremarkable. Muscle strength is normal. Anemia is common, and a markedly elevated erythrocyte sedimentation rate (ESR) is virtually always present. The ESR is usually > 50 mm/hr, and often > 100 mm/hr. Laboratory studies are also negative for rheumatoid factor, antinuclear antibodies, and elevated serum creatinine kinase. Some recommend temporal artery biopsy in all patients with PMR because of the high incidence of associated temporal arteritis (and the risk of blindness if not promptly treated with high dose corticosteroids). Patients with pure PMR (no symptoms or signs of temporal arteritis) can generally be treated with low-dose corticosteroids, with temporal artery biopsy reserved for those who subsequently develop symptoms.

If symptoms do not improve within one week, other diagnoses should be considered, such as **fibromyalgia** (also known as fibrositis). This disorder is similar to PMR in that the physical exam is usually unremarkable aside from tenderness, but fibromyalgia has multiple "trigger points," is most frequent in women aged 20 to 50, and the ESR is usually normal. **Osteoarthritis**, also known as degenerative joint disease (DJD), commonly occurs with aging and may be due to "wear and tear." It is characterized by loss of articular cartilage and bone remodeling and overgrowth. Patients experience a gradual onset of joint pain and stiffness that is usually made worse by activity and is relieved by rest. In contrast to rheumatoid arthritis (RA), DJD is not associated with systemic symptoms and the ESR and rheumatoid factor are normal. **Polymyositis** is a systemic disease of unknown etiology. In contrast to PMR, its main manifestation is bilateral weakness of proximal muscles, especially of the limbs. The disease is called dermatomyositis when it is associated with characteristic skin manifestations, such as purplish flushing of the eyelids, periorbital edema, and a red rash of the face, neck, shoulders, and torso. Dermatomyositis is associated with occult malignancy, such as ovarian cancer. Regardless of skin involvement, serum creatinine kinase (a muscle enzyme) is elevated. However, muscle biopsy is the only specific diagnostic test. **Rheumatoid arthritis** (RA) is a systemic inflammatory disease, likely autoimmune in nature. Systemic symptoms include malaise, fever, and weight loss. Like DJD, the onset of RA is insidious. Unlike DJD, the onset of RA is more often in women under age 40, stiffness is worse in the morning or with inactivity, and there are many extra-articular manifestations, such as subcutaneous nodules, pleural effusions, pericarditis, and vasculitis. Rheumatoid factor (RF) is positive in about 85% of patients, and anti-nuclear antibodies (ANA) are found in about 15%. Patients with classic RA may have negative tests for RF **(seronegative RA)** and are immunogenetically distinct from those that test positive for RF (seropositive RA). Seronegative RA tends to have a better articular prognosis and high titers of RF tend to correlate with more severe disease.

Ferri, 3rd ed., pp 776-80, 790-91.
Tierney, 38th ed., pp 798, 805-06, 817, 821-22.

21

(Block 1: Item 21)

(B)

Benign prostatic hyperplasia (BPH) is a nearly ubiquitous age-related disorder, and it causes urinary tract outflow obstruction in most men by the time they are 75 years old. Hyperplasia in BPH begins in the glandular tissue surrounding the urethra, thus causing outflow obstruction. This is in contrast to **prostate cancer**, which usually begins in the periphery and often does not cause symptoms until it is quite advanced. Obstructive symptoms of BPH include decreased force and caliber of the urinary stream, dribbling, urinary hesitancy, and nocturia. Hematuria may occur, although bladder cancer must be ruled out if it does. Obstruction causes bladder muscle hypertrophy, which results in bladder instability, urinary frequency, and incomplete bladder emptying. This leads to urinary retention, which predisposes to infection and can result in hydronephrosis and renal failure. Rectal examination classically reveals a uniformly enlarged prostate. Focal areas of induration may be found; further evaluation of these with transrectal ultrasound and possible biopsy is indicated to rule out cancer. Abdominal examination may reveal a distended bladder. Urinalysis may be normal or may indicate infection or hematuria, and serum creatinine should be checked to evaluate renal function. Prostatic-specific antigen (PSA) may be elevated in BPH as well as in prostate cancer. Insertion of a Foley catheter or bladder ultrasound often reveals a large residual volume (more than 100 mL is abnormal). Uroflowmetry (measurement of urine flow rate) can be used to demonstrate a decreased urinary peak flow rate. Treatment options include "watchful waiting", medications, and surgery. α_1 blockade with agents such as terazosin (Hytrin) and doxazosin (Cardura) improve symptoms by inhibiting prostatic smooth muscle contraction, though orthostatic hypotension may be common side effect. Finasteride decreases intraprostatic dihydrotestosterone (DHT) levels by inhibiting 5-α-reductase, which converts testosterone to DHT. This drug can decrease the size of the prostate and improve the symptoms of BPH. (Note that many commonly used drugs can exacerbate urinary outflow obstruction: anti-cholinergics, anti-depressants, and alpha-agonists in over-the-counter decongestants.) Transurethral resection of the prostate (TURP) is effective and has a low mortality rate, but there is a risk for postoperative sexual dysfunction. Other surgical options include thermotherapy with lasers, microwave, radiofrequency or high intensity focused ultrasound.

Acute prostatitis typically occurs in younger patients and is usually caused by *E. coli* or pseudomonas species ascending up the urethra with a resultant reflux of infected urine into the prostatic ducts. Symptoms and signs include suprapubic, perineal, or sacral pain, fever, dysuria, and sometimes urinary retention due to prostatic swelling. Rectal exam reveals a warm, tender, and boggy prostate. Urinalysis shows pyuria, bacteruria, and often hematuria. The offending bacterium will grow in urine culture. Complete blood count demonstrates an elevated white cell count with a left shift. **Neurogenic (neuropathic) bladder** results from damage to the spinal cord's micturition center at S2-S4, which is primarily responsible for the innervation of the bladder. Damage is most commonly due to trauma, and may occur at or above this spinal cord level. Lesions above S2-S4 are upper motor neuron (spastic) lesions that result in loss of control by higher centers and cause urinary retention. A lesion involving S2-S4 is a lower motor neuron (flaccid) lesion which results in inadequate bladder muscle contraction and, again, urinary retention. Clinically, neurogenic bladder can mimic obstruction, but there are usually other neurologic deficits associated with the responsible lesion. Urodynamic testing, which measures bladder pressure, may be needed to make the diagnosis. **Prostate cancer** is the most common cancer in American men (aside from skin cancer) and results in significant mortality. However, its incidence is far greater than its clinical significance, since the majority of all men have evidence of the disease at autopsy. The diagnosis is usually made in asymptomatic men who are found to have nodules or areas of induration on rectal examination. Patients may also present with back pain or pathologic fractures due to metastatic disease. PSA is useful in screening men for prostate cancer if used in adjunct with clinical exam of the prostate. In 1998, 70% of patients with detected cancer had an elevated or rising PSA along with a normal rectal exam. PSA is also useful for monitoring the recurrence of prostate cancer after treatment. **Urethral strictures** can present with the same symptoms as BPH, and can also result in urinary retention. They are usually due to prior instrumentation (e.g., Foley), and may also result from external trauma or inflammatory processes such as gonorrhea. Urethral strictures are not associated with an abnormal prostate exam. However, they will likely prevent the passage of a Foley.

Fauci, 14th ed., pp 41-42.
Goroll, 3rd ed., pp 705-07.
Tierney, 38th ed., pp 903, 915-20.
Way, 10th ed., pp 926-27, 962-64.

22

(Block 1: Item 22)

(B)

Traumatic crush injuries can cause rhabdomyolysis (muscle breakdown). Crush injuries are characterized by massive swelling (with influx of fluid into necrotic muscle) and skin and soft tissue ecchymoses; hypovolemic shock may also result. Necrotic muscle releases large amounts of myoglobin, which is freely filtered by the glomerulus. Myoglobin is reabsorbed by the tubules and can causes direct damage to them, resulting in acute tubular necrosis (ATN). 30% of rhabdomyolysis cases are complicated by myoglobinuric acute renal failure (ARF). Rhabdomyolysis can also occur after seizures or from lying unconscious all night on the sidewalk after drinking too much alcohol.

Prevention is the best treatment of ARF. Examples are aggressive hydration after surgery, major trauma, or burns; and avoidance or dosage adjustment of nephrotoxic drugs. Once a patient has ARF, care should be taken to avoid volume overload, hyperkalemia, and other electrolyte imbalances. Dialysis may be required for hyperkalemia, volume overload unresponsive to diuresis, severe acidosis, and uremic complications such as seizures or encephalopathy. Specific treatment for ARF secondary to myoglobinuria must address hypovolemia first; aggressive volume resuscitation should be instituted. Two to three liters of saline per hour are often required during the initial management, and 300 to 500 ml/h is necessary once hemodynamic stability has been achieved. Failure to provide adequate volume replacement is probably the most frequent error made in the management of rhabdomyolysis. Assessment of volume status often requires central venous or pulmonary artery pressure monitoring.

Therapy aimed at preventing the onset of ARF in rhabdomyolysis is controversial. Clinical studies suggest that alkaline diuresis (NOT **administration of hydrochloric acid until urine pH is 4.0**) is effective in preventing ARF in myoglobinuria. It is clear that increased urine volume is beneficial, and its alkalinization with bicarbonate probably adds to the beneficial effect of high urine flow. Likewise, the role of **mannitol diuresis** is controversial. It may reduce renal tubular oxygen consumption by reducing sodium resorption, which can reduce renal ischemic damage. Caution should be used in administering mannitol because an osmotic diuresis without adequate volume replacement might worsen hypovolemia. Some suggest that mannitol be added to the treatment regimen at a dose of 25 g every 6h. These measures are continued until myoglobinuria has resolved, unless volume overload limits intravenous fluid or serum osmolality limits mannitol administration. If there is no response in urine output to these measures, then furosemide is administered until a diuresis occurs.

Low, renal dose **dopamine** (1.0-5.0 mcg/kg/min, **continuous infusion**) has been widely used to treat ARF. Dopamine in these dosages is a potent vasodilator, which increases renal blood flow in the setting of ARF. In this scenario, the patient's ARF is largely due to rhabdomyolysis, not hypovolemia. Increasing blood flow to the kidneys will not combat the myoglobinuria. In addition, most clinical studies have failed to show that dopamine improves the recovery or mortality rates in ARF. Current recommendations for dopamine favor its use in ARF patients with congestive heart failure.

CT scanning is the standard imaging technique for quickly and accurately defining soft-tissue and bone abnormalities. **Oral and IV contrast** can be directly nephrotoxic (via intrarenal vasoconstriction) and would only "add insult to injury." Plain films (X-rays) are often obtained in the emergency room while the patient is being stabilized. If plain films are negative, and clinical suspicion of fracture remains high, a CT scan may be obtained once the patient is stable. Emergency **arteriography (angiography)** may be indicated for the evaluation of damage to peripheral vessels after trauma (but has the same concerns as IV contrast). Physical signs of arterial insufficiency (pallor, absent pulses) help determine the need for arteriography, although stabilization of the patient takes precedence over evaluating a limb.

Fauci, 14th ed., pp 1507, 1511-13.
Tierney, 38th ed., pp 867-70.
Schwartz, 4th ed., pp 170, 174, 741.
http://www.medstudents.com.br/terin/terin3.htm

23

(Block 1: Item 23)

(A)

Herpes zoster, also known as shingles, is a vesicular eruption caused by the reactivation of the varicella-zoster virus (human herpesvirus 3). The virus remains dormant in the cranial or dorsal root ganglion until reactivation, when it spreads along the cutaneous nerve giving rise to the characteristic distribution involving one dermatome. Although most patients with localized zoster are not immunosuppressed, states of immunosuppression such as HIV infection or non-Hodgkin's lymphoma are associated with zoster, presumably because of waning immunosurveillance of the dormant virus. Zoster usually affects adults and rarely occurs more than once in a given patient. The face (any of the 3 branches of the trigeminal nerve—in this patient it is in the distribution of V1) and the trunk are most commonly affected. Pain usually precedes the eruption, which consists of grouped vesicles distributed unilaterally in a dermatome. A Tzanck smear may be performed to confirm the diagnosis. Immunocompetent hosts may be treated with oral antivirals such as acyclovir or famciclovir. Patients over age 55 should receive oral antiviral treatment because they are more likely to develop postherpetic neuralgia (pain in the distribution of a nerve) as a complication. Treatment reduces this common complication of varicella zoster. However, oral antiviral therapy is effective in reducing postherpetic neuralgia only if initiated early in the course of infection (i.e. while vesicles are present). Systemic corticosteroids may minimize acute disease and do not predispose to dissemination in immunocompetent hosts. Immunosuppressed hosts (AIDS, transplant recipients, cancer patients) and immunocompetent patients at risk such as pregnant women and premature infants should be treated with intravenous or oral acyclovir, since VZV infections can be life-threatening.

Impetigo is a contagious skin infection caused by *Staphylococcus aureus* or group A beta-hemolytic streptococci. It typically occurs on the face of children, beginning as a superficial vesicle which ruptures and forms the classic honey-yellow crust. Gram stain and culture of the lesions confirm the diagnosis. **Pyoderma gangrenosum** is a non-infective skin disorder that causes chronic ulcers and high fever. The skin lesions may initially be nodules, but they quickly form ulcers that often have a bluish margin. Pyoderma gangrenosum is associated with ulcerative colitis and several immune disorders. **Syphilis**, which is caused by the spirochete *Treponema pallidum*, has a variety of manifestations including several skin lesions. Primary syphilis is characterized by a painless chancre (ulcer) which occurs at the site of inoculation (typically the genitalia). If untreated, the patient may develop secondary syphilis, which presents with fever and pink macular rash involving the genitalia, soles, palms, face, and trunk. After the roseola of secondary syphilis resolves, papular and papulosquamous lesions can develop. The hallmark of papular syphilis is the condyloma latum—a broad, flat papule or plaque located in the folds of moist skin, especially around the anus and genitalia. Tertiary syphilis is characterized by cardiovascular, neurologic, and skin manifestations.

The classic cutaneous lesion of tertiary syphilis is the gumma, which is a chronic granuloma that forms a papule or nodule, which can break down and ulcerate. Gummas are usually found on the skin and mucous membranes, but may involve any organ. **Systemic lupus erythematosus** (SLE) is an inflammatory autoimmune disorder that can involve various organs. Skin lesions include the characteristic "butterfly" rash, disc-like plaques on the face or scalp (discoid lupus), widespread maculopapular rash, and infarcts due to vasculitis that especially affects the hands and nail folds.

Tierney, 38th ed., pp 139-40, 143.
duVivier, 2nd ed., pp 11.14-11.17, 12.5-12.7, 16.18-16.19, 19.2-19.6.

24

(Block 1: Item 24)

(A)

Acute cystitis, or infection of the bladder, is the classic lower urinary tract infection (UTI). It typically presents with urinary frequency, urgency, dysuria, and suprapubic tenderness. Urinalysis shows pyuria, bacteriuria, and often hematuria. UTIs acquired outside of the hospital are generally caused by gram negative rods, such as *E. coli*, that are normally found in the gastrointestinal tract. Most UTIs are the result of **ascending infection from the urethra.** Women are particularly prone to UTIs because the female urethra is shorter than that of the male, and the vaginal introitus can become colonized with the offending bacteria. Sexual intercourse can be a precipitating factor for UTI, presumably because it facilitates the spread of organisms from the perineum to the vagina and urethra. Bacteriuria is significantly increased after 30% of intercourse episodes. The risk of UTI is further increased by the use of diaphragms and spermicidal jelly because they alter the normal vaginal bacterial flora. Women are also encouraged to wipe from front to back to help prevent UTI's. In contrast, the use of tampons and menarche are not risk factors for UTI. Prophylactic antibiotics should be considered for women who have more than 3 episodes of cystitis per year. These antibiotics can be taken regularly or at the time of intercourse.

Pyelonephritis occurs when the UTI ascends to involve the kidney parenchyma or renal pelvis. Findings include those for cystitis as well as fever, shaking chills, flank pain, and costovertebral angle tenderness. Pyelonephritis is usually caused by bacteria that ascend from the bladder via the ureters. The exception is *S. aureus*, which more commonly reaches the kidneys by the **hematogenous route**, from a source outside the urinary tract such as an abscess. Pelvic inflammatory disease (PID) generally refers to infection of the fallopian tubes (salpingitis), but can also include endometritis (infection of the uterine lining). PID is most commonly caused by chlamydia or gonorrhea, which can **ascend from the lower genital tract** if an infection there (e.g., urethritis, cervicitis) is not treated. PID can result in infertility, chronic pelvic pain, and an increased risk of ectopic pregnancy.

Benson, 1st ed., pp 170-73.
Goroll, 3rd ed., pp 681-82.
Tierney, 38th ed., pp 899-901.

25

(Block 1: Item 25)

(C)

Supracondylar fractures of the humerus occur frequently in children. Hyperextension at the elbow can cause an undisplaced (bone cortices remain aligned) fracture, while elbow hyperextension with superimposed rotation is more likely to cause a displaced (cortices knocked out of alignment) fracture. Because the displaced bone frequently compromises the vasculature, supracondylar fractures of the humerus can lead to compartment syndrome; this complication occurs when increased pressure in a closed fascial space results in compromised circulation and function. It can develop after fracture with subsequent hemorrhage and edema, crush injury, or electrical burns. The two classic fractures that can be complicated by compartment syndrome are supracondylar fractures of the humerus in children and tibial fractures. Increased pressure causes ischemia and ischemia for more than 6-8 hours results in death of nerve and muscle. This can cause Volkmann's contracture—forearm flexors undergo necrosis and are replaced by scar, leaving the wrist in flexion and the fingers clawed (thankfully with no associated nerve injury). In the case of compartment syndrome after a humeral fracture, the patient has a tense and swollen medial forearm (the flexor compartment), forearm weakness and anesthesia, and pain with wrist and finger extension (which stretches the involved muscles). Remember to look for the six P's of arterial insufficiency: pain, pallor, pulselessness, paresthesia, paralysis, and poikilothermia (cold). However, compartment syndrome can develop in the presence of pulses, since the pressure may be high enough to cause muscle and nerve ischemia without occluding a major artery. The diagnosis can be made clinically or by directly measuring the intracompartmental pressure with a catheter; pressures above 30-40 mm Hg may require intervention. The treatment of compartment syndrome is **emergent fasciotomy**, which involves opening the skin and fascia to decompress the compartment. When compartment syndrome is due to bleeding, or if there are signs of ischemia regardless of the presence compartment syndrome, arterial supply must be restored. Arteriography and **surgical exploration** may be required to identify and repair damaged vessels.

After elevated pressures are reduced and arterial flow is restored, or if these complications do not occur, displaced supracondylar fractures must be reduced (restored to alignment). Most cases can be treated with **closed reduction** under general anesthesia, by manipulating the distal fragment back into place. If the displacement is severe, another technique must be implemented. **Traction** may be used, or pins may be placed across the fracture percutaneously with fluoroscopic guidance after which the elbow is splinted. **Open reduction** is not generally required and introduces risk of infection. Open reduction is usually only indicated for intraarticular fractures, after a failed closed reduction, and in a setting of multiple trauma.

In undisplaced supracondylar fractures, closed reduction is indicated if angulation of the fracture exceeds 20 degrees. After reduction, or if reduction is not necessary, the arm should be casted or splinted. Regardless of fracture type and required treatment, the patient should be given **analgesics** for pain control.

Blackbourne, 2nd ed., p 650.
Way, 10th ed., pp 1063, 1075-76.

26

(Block 1: Item 26)

(C)

Hepatocellular carcinoma (HCC, **hepatoma**) develops in about 30% of patients with cirrhosis from any cause. Physical signs of cirrhosis may include jaundice, palmar erythema (EtOH abuse), spider angiomata, ecchymoses, caput medusae (dilated periumbilical veins), increased pigmentation, scleral icterus, fetor hepaticus, male gynecomastia, small nodular liver, ascites, hemorrhoids, and guaiac-positive stool. A long lists of diseases may progress to cirrhosis—EtOH abuse, secondary biliary cirrhosis, drugs, hepatic congestion, primary biliary cirrhosis, infiltrative diseases, chronic active hepatitis (viral or autoimmune), Wilson's disease, and α-1-antitrypsin deficiency, to name a few. In this asymptomatic patient, spider angiomata, atrophic testes, and a small, shrunken liver point to chronic cirrhosis; the additional findings of increased skin pigmentation and cardiac enlargement with a S3 suggest hemochromatosis as the cause. As a result of increased deposition of hemosiderin in organs, hemochromatosis can also cause arthropathy, cardiac enlargement with failure and conduction defects, "bronze diabetes", and male impotence. HCC (hepatoma) is an unfortunate consequence in 15-20% of patients with hemochromatosis. It is four times more common in men than women and is usually coexistent with a cirrhotic liver. Unfortunately, patients with multifocal disease and concomitant cirrhosis are not candidates for surgical resection; liver transplantation and chemoembolization via the hepatic artery are options for some HCC patients.

Wernicke's encephalopathy manifests itself as sixth nerve palsy and ataxia and is most often caused by thiamine deficiency. It is usually the result of chronic alcoholism. **Cerebellar degeneration** is a rare syndrome of gait ataxia and nystagmus also associated with chronic alcoholism. **Hepatic vein thrombosis** (Budd-Chiari syndrome) results in ascites and a grossly enlarged liver (associated with occlusion of the hepatic veins or IVC) usually without signs and symptoms of heart failure. It is not a consequence of cirrhosis but usually of hypercoagulable states, myeloproliferative syndromes, or HCC (hepatoma). Hepatorenal syndrome causing **renal failure** is an uncommon complication in patients with end-stage liver disease and ascites, and presents with symptoms of azotemia, oliguria, hyponatremia, low urinary sodium, and hypotension. Etiology is unknown, and treatment is usually ineffective.

Fauci, 14th ed., pp 1709, 2150-51, 2504.
Ferri, 3rd ed., pp 364-65.

27

(Block 1: Item 27)

(E)

Hypoglycemia (< 30 mg/dL in a full-term baby) occurs in up to 40% of neonates of diabetic mothers; untreated hypoglycemia can cause seizures, apnea, and cyanosis leading to irreversible brain damage. An Apgar score of 7 in this question indicates a moderately depressed infant; this information, combined with the fact that the mother is a diabetic in poor control, should lead to immediate determination of **serum glucose levels** in the neonate. Infants of diabetic mothers also have higher rates of perinatal death, intrauterine growth restriction and congenital malformations. As with this child, macrosomia is a major risk in diabetic pregnancies; the macrosomic infant is more likely to have delayed organ development.

Determination of blood group and Rh as well as hematocrit is routinely done post-delivery to detect antibody-mediated blood group abnormalities. **Determination of pH** is only done if hypoxia is suspected in the neonate. **Measurement of serum bilirubin** is used to evaluate jaundice in a neonate. Obtaining serum glucose should take precedence in the case of a mother with poorly controlled Type I diabetes mellitus.

DeCherney, 8th ed., pp 377-78.

28

(Block 1: Item 28)

(D)

The diagnosis of **uterine atony** is made by palpating the uterus and finding "the fundus...soft and boggy". Uterine atony can cause postpartum hemorrhage (> 500 mL in a vaginal delivery, > 1000 mL in a cesarean section). Postpartum hemorrhage is the third leading cause for maternal death in the USA. Uterine atony, or failure of the myometrium to contract after delivery, causes 50% of cases of postpartum hemorrhage; multiparous patients, patients with a history of atony, and patients with uterine abnormalities or fibroids are at particular risk. It is more common with oxytocin augmentation and prolonged labor, as in this question. Treatment of uterine atony consists of Pitocin IV accompanied by vigorous uterine massage. If this is unsuccessful, the next step is methylergonovine; PGF-2α is then given directly into the uterine musculature if bleeding persists. Persistent, life-threatening hemorrhage may require ligation of uterine arteries or hysterectomy.

Lacerations cause 20% of postpartum hemorrhage cases and should be suspected if there is bleeding when the uterus is firm and well contracted. **Cervical lacerations** are commonly the results of rapid dilation during the first stage of labor or commencement of the second stage of labor without complete dilation of the cervix. **Retained placental tissue** causes 5-10% of postpartum hemorrhages, emphasizing the importance of inspecting the placenta thoroughly. Occasionally retained placenta and fetal membranes can causes endomyometritis. **Disseminated intravascular coagulation (DIC)** is associated with preeclampsia, sepsis, abruptio placentae, retained dead fetus, and amniotic fluid embolus; it is unusual in an otherwise normal delivery. This dreaded complication can present with excessive bleeding (hemorrhage, oozing at IV sites, petechiae), hypotension, and abnormal coagulation studies (elevated PT, D-dimer). An **inverted uterus** occurs in 1 of 25,000 deliveries; it can happen when there is excessive traction on the cord in the third stage of labor. Fundal implantation of the placenta, uterine atony, and placenta accreta are also risk factors for uterine inversion. Often the diagnosis is made when delivery of placenta includes the fundus of the uterus. Treatment is manual reinversion of the uterus; nitroglycerin may be given to aid relaxation of the uterus.

DeCherney, 8th ed., pp 574-75.

29

(Block 1: Item 29)

(B)

Fibroadenoma is the most common breast mass in women under 30. It is classically described as a firm, nontender, round, rubbery, mobile 1-5 cm mass. 10-15% of patients have multiple fibroadenomas in one or both breasts. After diagnosis by needle biopsy or cytologic examination, no treatment is necessary; some women opt for excisional biopsy.

Fat necrosis of the breast is uncommon. It is thought to be secondary to trauma and presents with a firm mass that can have associated skin or nipple retraction. It resolves without treatment, but cannot be distinguished from cancer without biopsy. **Fibrocystic changes** are very common and are associated with pain, tenderness, and irregular thickenings that change with the menstrual cycle. There are usually multiple sites in both breasts. **Intraductal carcinoma** may or may not be associated with a mass. A cancerous mass, if present, is more often hard, irregular, and non-mobile. Carcinoma is rare in women under 25. **Intraductal papilloma** is a benign lesion that may or may not be associated with a mass, but is often associated with spontaneous serous or serosanguinous nipple discharge. Every breast mass should be worked up; one approach might first start with an ultrasound of the mass (to determine if it is cystic or solid) and then proceed to fine needle aspiration (FNA) of the mass. The results of the FNA would guide subsequent diagnostics or treatment.

DeCherney, 8th ed., pp 1118-26.

30

(Block 1: Item 30)

(B)

Aplastic anemia is characterized by trilineage depletion of bone marrow precursor cells with subsequent pancytopenia. The anemia can be severe and is always associated with a decreased reticulocyte count. Bone marrow aspirate or biopsy is hypocellular with rare hematopoietic progenitors seen. Most cases are acquired from exposure to drugs, viruses, organic compounds, or irradiation. Chloramphenicol has a nasty reputation for causing both reversible and irreversible bone marrow suppression. Irreversible aplastic anemia occurs in 1/25,000-40,000 exposures to chloramphenicol. Although it is available as an 'over the counter' drug in Mexico, chloramphenicol is rarely used in the U.S.

This child does not have **anemia due to blood loss**, as that does not explain her reduction in platelets, leukocytes, and reticulocytes. **Aplastic crises in sickle cell disease** does not cause reduction in all three cell lineages; typically a viral infection (parvovirus B19) or folate deficiency leads to suppression of marrow erythroid precursors and causes a severe anemia with reticulocytopenia. **Infectious mononucleosis** usually causes an increase in lymphocyte number as well as lymphadenopathy and splenomegaly. **Viral-induced pancytopenia** is a possible answer, but, given the recent history of chloramphenicol exposure and the lack of a viral prodrome, it is far less likely.

Fauci, 14th ed., pp 672-75, 866.
Tierney, 38th ed., pp 497, 501-03, 1452.

31

(Block 1: Item 31)

(E)

The definition of **major depressive disorder** requires five of the following symptoms over a two-week period: (1) depressed or irritable mood, (2) diminished interest in activities, (3) significant weight loss without dieting, (4) insomnia or hypersomnia, (5) psychomotor agitation or retardation, (6) fatigue or loss of energy, (7) feelings of worthlessness or guilt, (8) diminished ability to concentrate, and (9) recurrent thoughts of death or suicidal ideation. One symptom must be either a depressed mood or the loss of interest or pleasure. All symptoms must demonstrate a change from previous functioning and cannot be secondary to a medical condition, substance abuse, or bereavement. A common mnemonic for these criteria is SIG E CAPS: **s**leep, **i**nterests, **g**uilt, **e**nergy, **c**oncentration, **a**ppetite, **p**sychomotor retardation/agitation, **s**uicidality.

Adjustment disorder with mixed disturbance of emotion and conduct requires the development of symptoms to be related to an identifiable psychosocial stressor and is a diagnosis of exclusion. Adjustment disorders usually develop within 3 months of the acute stressor and resolve within 6 months. **Anorexia nervosa** (AN) is an eating disorder that can often present concurrently with major depressive disorder. DSM-IV criteria for AN include refusal to maintain body weight at greater than 85% of ideal, intense fear of "being fat," preoccupation with body size and shape, denial of the medical risks of low weight, and a disproportionate influence of body weight on personal worth. For females, amenorrhea is also a diagnostic criterion. Orthostatic hypotension and bradycardia are typical physical signs of AN. **Attention-deficit/hyperactivity disorder** is diagnosed in children who display inattention, hyperactivity, and impulsivity; these children usually display symptoms consistent with ADHD before age 7. **Dysthymic disorder** requires a depressed mood on most days for at least 2 years, although children and adolescents can be diagnosed if irritable or depressed for 1 year.

Goldman, 4th ed., pp 250, 302, 356.

32

(Block 1 Item 32)

(D)

This patient has a hypochromic, microcytic (MCV < 85 fL) anemia with moderate poikilocytosis (fragmented RBCs). RBC fragmentation may result from trauma through her stenotic aortic valve. Her cardiac symptoms are exacerbated by her anemia (pallor), which can cause angina and heart failure (SOB, JVD, and rales) in patients with preexisting heart disease. The differential diagnosis for microcytic anemias includes iron deficiency, thalassemia, lead poisoning, vitamin B_6 deficiency, anemia of chronic disease and sideroblastic anemia. **Iron deficiency** is by far the most common cause of microcytic anemia and blood loss is the most important cause in adults. In this case, we know the patient has occult blood loss in her stool.

Anemia of chronic disease (ACD) can also cause a microcytic (normal to mild), hypochromic anemia, but it is usually associated with inflammatory diseases, chronic infections, cancer, and liver disease. ACD can be misdiagnosed as an iron deficiency anemia; it is important to look at the iron studies because ACD differs from iron deficiency only in a low TIBC (total iron-binding capacity) value. Since this patient has a near normal erythrocyte sedimentation rate and no history of infection, malignancy, or liver disease, it is not a likely diagnosis. **Autoimmune hemolytic anemia** usually follows a viral infection and includes elevated bilirubin, elevated reticulocyte count, and normal MCV. **Folate deficiency anemia** has an increased MCV. **Microangiopathic hemolytic anemia** can be caused by a panoply of disorders (TTP, HUS, DIC, metastatic adenocarcinoma, vasculitis, and valve hemolysis). Laboratory findings show elevated bilirubin, elevated reticulocyte count, normal MCV, and multiple erythrocyte fragments (schistocytes, helmet cells). This patient probably has a degree of chronic microangiopathic hemolytic anemia secondary to her severely narrowed aortic value; this may contribute to the iron deficiency anemia and cause low-grade hemoglobinuria.

Hoffman, 2nd ed., pp 474, 480, 506-11, 1850, 1885.

33

(Block 1: Item 33)

(D)

This patient has the classic signs of meningitis: fever, stiff neck, and flu-like symptoms. The fact that he is difficult to wake and had an acute onset of symptoms suggests bacterial meningoencephalitis. He also has a purpuric rash over his extremities and vital signs consistent with septic shock, suggesting coexistent meningococcemia (a fulminant form of septicemia due to *Neisseria meningitidis*). ***Neisseria meningitidis*** is the cause of epidemic meningitis and is found most often in children and young adults, especially those living in dormitories, barracks, or other close quarters (polysaccharide vaccines are available). CSF of a patient with community-acquired purulent meningitis would show 200-20,000 WBC/μL, low glucose, and high protein with a markedly elevated opening pressure. Gram stain of the CSF may reveal Gram-negative intracellular and extracellular diplococci. Blood cultures should be obtained and IV antimicrobials started immediately (penicillin G or ceftriaxone). Signs of cerebral edema and increased intracranial pressure may prompt use of dexamethasone. Remember that household member of patients with meningococcal meningitis should be given rifampin or fluoroquinolone prophylaxis.

Coxsackievirus B and **Echovirus** (enteroviruses) can cause viral meningitis in children and young adults; viral (aseptic) meningitis is more benign than purulent meningitis in immunocompetent adults. Echovirus and rickettsial infection may also produce a petechial rash. ***Haemophilus influenzae*** typically causes meningitis (although uncommon since the advent of the *H. Influenzae* vaccine) in children under 2 years of age and is a rare cause of meningitis in adults; ***Streptococcus pneumonia*** is the most common etiological agent for bacterial meningitis in adults; pneumococcal meningitis does not produce a rash and neurologic abnormalities are often more prominent.

Fauci, 14th ed., pp 2420-21, 2440.

34

(Block 1: Item 34)

(E)

Anterior chest trauma combined with hypotension and distended neck veins and equal breath sounds = cardiac tamponade! Classic findings are decreasing arterial pressure, increasing central venous pressure, and distant heart sounds. The amount of fluid necessary to produce these changes can be as little as 200cc acutely; **pericardio-**

centesis is the correct procedure to perform. Since the patient has good breath sounds bilaterally, an **X-ray film of the chest** is not acutely necessary and may delay treatment. Likewise, **endotracheal intubation** is not indicated. An **ECG** will not add information to this clinical picture and again would delay treatment. **Insertion of a chest tube** is acutely indicated for a tension pneumothorax compromising cardiac output, which would be evident by hypotension, decreased or absent breath sounds on one side and distended neck veins (a late finding is tracheal deviation away from the injured side). This patient has good breath sounds bilaterally and no evidence of respiratory compromise so chest tube placement is unnecessary.

Fauci, 14th ed., pp 1336-37.

35

(Block 1: Item 35)

(A)

This patient has evidence of a stage I pressure (decubitus) ulcer. More than 95% of pressure ulcers develop in the lower half of the body, usually over bony prominences. Risk factors include immobility, age, poor nutrition, and moisture over the area. Preventive measures include frequent turning of bedridden patients. A **turning schedule** of once every 2 hours is standard. Use of **wet to dry dressings, whirlpool therapy, antibiotics or debridement** is not needed at this stage as the skin is only erythematous and there is no sign of infection or necrosis.

DeLisa, 3rd ed., pp 1057-1068.

36

(Block 1: Item 36)

(D)

The key information in this question is that the infant's stool is bulky, oily, and positive for fat. **Malabsorption** is characterized by loose and bulky stools, poor weight gain, and abdominal distention. Colitis, characterized by anemia or obvious blood in the stools, can occur. Allergic symptoms such as eczema or wheezing may also be a feature of malabsorption. Malabsorption is part of a larger differential for "failure to thrive", defined as persistent weight below the third percentile or falling off one's growth curve.

Absence of ganglia in the distal bowel, known as Hirschsprung's disease, typically presents with failure to pass meconium and abdominal distention. It does not cause fat malabsorption, nor would an **anatomic bowel obstruction**. Both **growth hormone deficiency** and **psychosocial neglect** can cause impaired growth in infants, but again would not cause increased fat in the stools. Gluten-induced enteropathy, carbohydrate malabsorption, and cystic fibrosis account for more than 90% of pediatric malabsorption cases.

Avery, 2nd ed., pp 485, 513-14.

37

(Block 1: Item 37)

(B)

Cystic fibrosis can present as a malabsorptive syndrome due to diminished pancreatic enzyme secretion. Because a **sweat chloride** test is easy, inexpensive, and virtually diagnostic of CF, it should be done in any infant with failure to thrive, steatorrhea, or malabsorption syndromes. A level greater than 60 mEq/L is considered abnormal. Other gastrointestinal manifestations of CF include bowel obstruction with rectal prolapse, diabetes, and hepatic cirrhosis. In the neonate, meconium ileus is pathognomonic for CF. In addition, all levels of the respiratory tract may be affected in CF; nasal polyps, opacification of the sinuses and sinusitis, and repeated bacterial pneumonias (90% of patients acquire *Pseudomonas aeruginosa*) are common.

Family counseling would be useful if psychosocial neglect were thought to be the cause of poor growth. A **serum hormone assay** would be helpful in determining if low thyroid hormone or growth hormone levels were causing poor growth. **Colon contrast studies** would be helpful in diagnosing celiac disease or an anatomic bowel obstruction, and **biopsy of the distal bowel** (showing absence of ganglia) would diagnose Hirschsprung's disease.

Avery, 2nd ed., pp 485, 513-14.

38

(Block 1: Item 38)

(C)

Over two-thirds of patients with lymphadenopathy in a primary care setting have non-specific or benign causes, and fewer than 1% have a malignancy. Generalized lymphadenopathy is more often associated with non-malignant causes, whereas regional lymphadenopathy, as in this case, is more commonly malignant. This patient has an enlarging, painless supraclavicular node, mediastinal lymphadenopathy and constitutional symptoms of fever and night sweats. These features point to **Hodgkin's disease (HD)**, which presents as painless lymph node enlargement, constitutional symptoms of fever and night sweats in 25%, and pruritus in 10% of patients. HD has a bimodal age distribution (15 to 34 years and over age 50). Symptoms of HD which have prognostic significance are (1) weight loss (> 10% in prior 6 months), (2) night sweats, and (3) fever. These compromise the "B" symptoms. Patients with no "B" symptoms have the "A" designation as part of their stage (i.e. Stage IA, Stage IIA, etc.). Patients with "B" symptoms have the "B" designation (i.e. Stage IB, IIB, etc.). Stage for stage, patients with "A" disease have a better prognosis than those with "B" disease. Pruritus and pain with alcohol ingestion are symptoms sometimes seen in HD but are neither diagnostic nor prognostic. Cough (due to lung involvement), superior vena cava (SVC) syndrome (due to extensive mediastinal involvement), or cord compression are symptoms associated with the direct mass effect of advanced disease.

Chronic lymphocytic leukemia has a median age of onset of 60 and usually presents with incidental lymphocytosis. **Drug reactions** can cause generalized lymphadenopathy, but we have no history of medications in this patient. **Infectious mononucleosis** usually presents with generalized or posterior cervical lymphadenopathy and pharyngitis. **Metastatic carcinoma** often presents with hard, immobile ("matted") nodes, not rubbery as in this case. **Sarcoidosis** classically involves hilar and paratracheal lymphadenopathy with pulmonary symptoms. **Systemic lupus erythematosus (SLE)** has other manifestations of disease including rash, joint pain, and splenomegaly, and is more common in young women. **Toxoplasmosis** (*Toxoplasma gondii*) usually presents with cervical lymphadenopathy in patients with a history of cat exposure and is unusual in immunocompetent persons. **Tuberculosis** can present as painless lymphadenopathy at cervical and supraclavicular sites; this is most common in HIV-infected patients. **Tularemia** (*Francisella tularensis*) is associated with fever, chills, headache, ulcerative skin lesions and tender lymphadenopathy.

Fauci, 14th ed., pp 346-47, 424, 708, 972, 1089, 1199, 1925.

39

(Block 1: Item 39)

(B)

Phenytoin and primidone are both **drugs** known to cause lymphadenopathy as an occasional adverse reaction. Phenytoin can also cause epigastric pain and headaches. The lymph node biopsy showing hyperplasia rules out malignancy and the patient's medication history makes drug reaction the most likely answer.

Fauci, 14th ed., pp 346-47, 424.

40

(Block 1: Item 40)

(C)

Cluster headaches usually affect middle-aged men and present with severe pain around one eye occurring nightly for several weeks. Ipsilateral nasal congestion or lacrimation is common, as is ptosis and myosis on the affected side. Spontaneous remissions occur, lasting from weeks to months, before another "cluster" of attacks occurs.

Acute or chronic sinusitis is often associated with facial pain over the maxillary or frontal sinuses and a history of respiratory tract infection. **Intracranial tumors** causing headache are progressive over time and usually cause neurologic deficits as well. **Meningoencephalitis** and **subarachnoid hemorrhage** preset with acute severe headache, signs of meningeal irritation and impairment of consciousness. **Migraines** are unilateral, throbbing headaches associated with nausea, vomiting, photophobia, and vision changes. **Pheochromocytoma** is very rare (less than 1% of hypertensive patients) and causes attacks of headache, sweating, and palpitations. **Post-traumatic headache** is a dull, constant ache associated with a history of trauma. **Temporal arteritis** is most common in elderly patients and presents with headache associated with myalgia and malaise and tenderness over the temporal artery. **Temporomandibular joint syndrome (TMJ)** presents with tenderness of muscles of mastication and face or head pain that is associated with jaw movement. It occurs in individuals with malocclusion or faulty dentures.

Tierney, 38th ed., pp 933, 936, 1102.

41

(Block 1: Item 41)

(F)

This is a classic presentation for a **migraine**: throbbing, unilateral pain associated with nausea, vomiting and photophobia. Focal neurologic disturbances including numbness, clumsiness, or weakness may occur. Onset is usually in adolescence or early adult life. Some patients describe triggers including foods (alcohol, chocolate), menstrual cycle, oral contraceptives, and stress. Rarely, patients may have a painless migraine in which the neurologic disturbances are the sole manifestation.

Tierney, 38th ed., pp 932-33.

42

(Block 1: Item 42)

(D)

Infectious mononucleosis is commonly caused by salivary transmission of the **Epstein-Barr virus** (human herpes virus 4). Mononucleosis typically presents in adolescents and young adults with pharyngitis, malaise, anorexia, myalgia and fever. Lymphadenopathy (usually posterior cervical and discrete, nonsuppurative, and slightly painful) and splenomegaly are common. Laboratory exam shows a lymphocytosis with dark, large, vacuolated lymphocytes. Hepatic enzymes are often elevated, and heterophil antibody tests are positive within four weeks of infection. Less commonly, infectious mononucleosis can cause hepatitis, central nervous system involvement (with painful mononeuropathies [Bell's palsy], aseptic meningitis, Guillain-Barre syndrome, and encephalitis), interstitial nephritis (with renal failure), pulmonary involvement, and myocarditis.

Acute leukemia may present with fever, bleeding, cytopenia, and blasts in peripheral blood; sore throat is not a presenting sign. **Folic acid or Vitamin B_{12} deficiency** causes a macrocytic anemia with hypersegmented neutrophils. **Anemia of chronic disease** and **iron deficiency** cause a microcytic anemia, which is not present. **Glucose 6-phosphate (G6PD) deficiency** and hereditary spherocytosis cause a hemolytic anemia.

Tierney, 38th ed., pp 511, 1262.

43

(Block 1: Item 43)

(A)

Patients with **acute leukemia** usually seek treatment because of bleeding, fatigue, or bone and joint pain. Cellulitis, pneumonia, and other infections due to neutropenia can also be presenting symptoms. Occasionally, very high circulating leukocyte numbers can present as headache, confusion, and dyspnea. Laboratory findings include pancytopenia with high numbers of circulating blasts in the periphery. None of the other answers adequately explain the patient's combination of pancytopenia, bleeding, and bone pain.

Tierney, 38th ed., pp 511-12.

44

(Block 1: Item 44)

(H)

Leiomyomata uteri, commonly known as "fibroids", are quite common, present in about 25% of reproductive age women. These benign smooth muscle neoplasms are usually asymptomatic, but can cause metrorrhagia (intermenstrual bleeding), menorrhagia (heavy or prolonged menstrual bleeding), pain, and infertility. Abnormal bleeding occurs in 30% of patients and is a common indication for hysterectomy in the U.S. Large fibroids can cause a feeling of heaviness or fullness in the pelvic area and occasionally pain. In 2-10% of patients, infertility is the presenting complaint. On bimanual exam most fibroids are felt as one or more smooth, firm masses distorting the normal uterine contour. Anemia may also be present.

The differential for uterine leiomyomas includes pregnancy, ovarian malignancy, tubo-ovarian abscess and endometriosis. In this patient **ectopic pregnancy** is unlikely since she is menstruating at regular intervals. **Corpus luteum cysts, dermoid cysts, and follicular cysts** are unlikely answers as they present as adnexal (ovarian) masses and do not usually cause menorrhagia. **Endometriosis** presents most commonly with pelvic pain and dysmenorrhea. **Granulosa cell tumors** of the ovary are associated with hyperestrogenism that causes precocious puberty in girls and postmenopausal bleeding in adult women. A **Sertoli-Leydig cell tumor** is a virilizing ovarian tumor that usually presents in the third decade. **Tubo-ovarian abscess** presents as a painful adnexal mass following pelvic infection.

DeCherney, 8th ed., pp 730-34, 774, 958-59.

45

(Block 1: Item 45)

(B)

Dermoid cysts are also known as benign cystic teratomas. They occur between the ages of 20 and 40 and are almost exclusively benign. These cysts are composed of well-differentiated tissues of ectodermal, mesodermal, and endodermal origin. They are often filled with sebaceous material, hair, and in 30-50% they contain teeth, making them visible on plain X-ray films of the abdomen. These tumors are treated with surgical resection. This patient's palpable adnexal mass combined with visible calcifications on X-ray makes dermoid cyst the likely diagnosis. Uterine leiomyomata can occasionally undergo calcific degeneration but there are no other signs of fibroids in this patient. Neither functional ovarian cysts nor ovarian carcinomas have associated calcifications visible on X-ray.

DeCherney, 8th ed., pp 732, 958.

46

(Block 1: Item 46)

(D)

An **endometrioma** is a solitary, non-neoplastic mass containing endometrial tissue and blood. Endometriosis is thought to have a prevalence of 10% in reproductive-age women. It is caused by the abnormal growth of endometrial tissue outside the uterus, most commonly on the peritoneal surfaces of the ovaries, cul-de-sac, bladder, and rarely in the lung, brain and other distant sites. Most women present with infertility and/or pelvic pain. Dyspareunia (pain with intercourse) is often present. A large implantation can cause a feeling of pelvic pressure, pain, and even bowel obstruction. Physical exam classically shows tender nodules in the posterior fornix, pain on uterine motion, tender adnexal masses (endometriomas) and, in severe cases, uterosacral nodularity and a fixed retroverted uterus. When an ovary is involved, a tender, fixed, adnexal mass may be palpated. Definitive diagnosis can only be made by direct visualization—remember, rust to dark brown "powder burns", "raspberry" or "mulberry" lesions, dense adhesions (as a result of reactive fibrosis), and "chocolate cysts" (thick, old, dark blood) may be seen. Treatment consists of hormonal suppressive therapy, surgery, or hysterectomy. Although endometrioma is the most likely diagnosis in this case, **neoplasms of the ovary** cannot be ruled out without surgical exploration. The differential also includes chronic pelvic inflammatory disease, recurrent acute salpingitis, hemorrhagic corpus luteum cyst, and ectopic pregnancy.

Fauci, 14th ed., p 2115.
DeCherney, 8th ed., pp 802-06.

47

(Block 1: Item 47)

(B)

Acute aortic dissection is classically described as an acute, severe, tearing pain in the chest and back. It is often interscapular and migrates as the dissection progresses. Hypertension is a predisposing factor in 70% of patients who present with dissection, usually men between the ages of 60 and 80 years. Aortic dissection is also a major cause of morbidity in patients with Marfan's syndrome, which is probably the case in this 37-year-old with a tall, lanky frame (6'8" tall and 190 lbs.). Marfan's syndrome is a connective tissue disorder that has widespread physical abnormalities. Patients with this syndrome present with disproportionate growth (arachnodactyly), joint hyper-extensibility, lens dislocation, and dilation of the aortic root. The defect in fibrillin, a structural component of elastin associated microfibrils, leads to disruption of collagen and elastin fibers in vessels and valves, thereby causing dilation, dissection and rupture of the aorta and prolapse of the valves. Cardiovascular abnormalities cause many fatalities in these patients. Physical findings with acute dissection may include loss of pulses, aortic regurgitation, pulmonary edema, hypertension or hypotension, and neurologic damage from carotid artery involvement. Chest X-ray may show a widened mediastinum, but ECG is usually normal. Definitive diagnosis is usually established with dynamic CT scanning, angiography, or transesophageal echocardiography (TEE).

The pain of **angina pectoris** (due to myocardial ischemia) is usually described as a sensation of pressure, squeezing, or heaviness in the anterior chest. **Aortic stenosis** and **hypertrophic cardiomyopathy** also cause this type of ischemic pain. **Myocardial infarction** produces similar pain with characteristic ECG changes. **Mitral valve prolapse** is usually painless. **Arthritis of the spine, cervical disc disease,** and **costochondritis** all cause recurrent pain that is persistent and aggravated by movement or direct pressure. An **aortic aneurysm** is a painless dilatation of the aorta, usually in the abdominal region that occurs as a result of atherosclerosis, infection, or injury. **Chronic constrictive pericardiopathy** results when the pericardium becomes scarred and restricted around the heart and interferes with ventricular filling. Signs and symptoms include weakness, fatigue, dyspnea, and jugular venous distention, but not pain. **Pericardial tamponade** causes symptoms similar to constrictive pericardiopathy. **Duodenal ulcer** and **hiatal hernia** cause epigastric pain that is burning or gnawing in character. **Esophageal spasm** may cause acute chest pain that radiates to the back or neck. It can be difficult to distinguish from myocardial ischemia, but only lasts for seconds to minutes and may occur with dysphagia. **Herpes zoster** causes cutaneous pain along dermatomal lines and is most often associated with a rash in that distribution. **Lung disease** typically causes symptoms of dyspnea or orthopnea. Pain, if present, is usually pleuritic.

Fauci, 14th ed., pp 58-59, 1339, 1394-96, 1591-92, 1601.

48

(Block 1: Item 48)

(W)

Pulmonary embolism occurs when a blood clot travels through the vasculature and obstructs the pulmonary vascular bed. Most emboli come from the deep veins of the legs or pelvis. Factors predisposing to the development of PE include immobilization, surgery, malignancy, chronic disease states (COPD, diabetes, CHF), oral contraceptive use, obesity, and coagulation disorders (protein C deficiency, protein S deficiency, Factor V Leiden, antithrombin III deficiency, lupus anticoagulant, polycythemia vera, dysfibrinogenemia, paroxysmal nocturnal hemoglobinuria). The most common symptom of pulmonary embolism is dyspnea, although pleuritic chest pain and hemoptysis may be present. Physical exam may show tachypnea, fever, diaphoresis, tachycardia, hypotension, and, perhaps, evidence for a deep venous thrombosis (DVT). With a large embolus, the pulmonary artery pressure may increase enough to cause right heart failure and findings of right heart strain on ECG. Chest X-ray may be completely normal. Ventilation-perfusion scanning combined with clinical suspicion is essential for diagnosis in the case of suspected PE; helical (spiral) CT and magnetic resonance angiography (MRA) are also employed at centers that have these diagnostic technologies available. Therapy involves anticoagulation with IV heparin and warfarin; heparin is usually stopped after 4-7 days of concomitant therapy with warfarin. Activated partial thromboplastin time (APTT), INR, and platelet count should be monitored. Massive PE may require thrombolytic therapy or emergent surgical embolectomy.

Fauci, 14th ed., pp 1469-71.
Ferri, 3rd ed., p 614.

49

(Block 1: Item 49)

(D, E, F, I) not (D, E, F, G)

As of the date of this publication, there was an error in the original answer published by the NBME.

A young man who has received no immunizations since the age of 5 and who is entering the medical profession should receive (1) Td **(tetanus-diphtheria toxoid)**. This is the form used in adults and children over 7; it is less likely to produce a local reaction than DTP. It is recommended that adults receive a booster every 10 years to prevent against tetanus and diphtheria. He should also receive (2) **hepatitis B vaccine**. Universal vaccination of children against Hep B is now recommended, with doses at birth, 1 and 6 months, and a booster at 12 years. All health care personnel should be vaccinated due to their exposure to blood products. He should receive an annual (3) **influenza vaccine**. Although usually recommended for elderly or chronically ill patients, healthy adults who are in contact with patients should be vaccinated annually to prevent transmission of the disease. Finally, this man needs (4) **MMR (measles-mumps-rubella vaccine)**. In 1989 there was a resurgence of measles in the U.S. partially due to MMR vaccine failure. It is recommended that anyone entering college, traveling abroad, or entering a health care job be vaccinated as an adult, unless they were born before 1957 or have documented measles history or immunity.

Haemophilus influenzae **Type b (Hib) vaccine** is given to infants at 2,4 and 6 months with a booster at 1 year. Children over age 2 who have not been vaccinated do not need to be, unless they have sickle cell anemia or asplenia. **Hepatitis B immune globulin** is given as postexposure prophylaxis in children born to Hepatitis B surface antigen positive mothers and in exposed adults. **Oral poliovirus (OPV)** replicates in the gut and can rarely cause polio. It should never be given to immunodeficient persons, unvaccinated adults, or health care workers. In these cases inactivated virus (IPV) should be used. **Pneumococcal vaccine** is recommended for the elderly, the chronically ill, and those who are asplenic.

Hay, 13th ed., pp 238-51.
Fauci, 14th ed., pp 762-65.

50

(Block 1: Item 50)

(A, B, D, G)

A six-month old child who has not had immunizations should be started immediately with **DTP (Diphtheria-tetanus-pertussis vaccine), *Haemophilus influenzae*** **type b (Hib)**, **Hepatitis B vaccine** and **OPV**. DTP should be given at 6, 8, and 10 months with a booster at 16 months. The booster should be DTaP (acellular pertussis) in children > 15 months of age. Hib should be given at 6, 8, and 10 months with a booster at 16 months. Hep B vaccine should be given at 6, 7, and 10-12 months with a booster at 12 years. OPV should be given at 6, 8, 16 months with a booster at 4-6 years.

Hay, 13th ed., pp 238-51.

51

(Block 2: Item 1)

(A)

Benign positional vertigo is a type of transient vertigo that follows changes in head position. Dizziness on lying down and getting up is a typical complaint. True "benign positional vertigo" is peripheral in origin. Unlike central nervous system disorders, peripheral lesions are characterized by a latency period of several seconds following positional change before symptoms develop. Symptoms usually occur in clusters and may continue for several days. Fatigable, horizontal nystagmus also supports the diagnosis of benign positional vertigo; the associated nystagmus with central lesions (e.g., brain stem vascular disease, arteriovenous malformations, tumors of the brainstem and the cerebellum, multiple sclerosis, and vertebrobasilar migraine) is usually nonfatigable, vertical in orientation, and unsuppressed by visual fixation. Treatment options for benign positional vertigo include head positioning physical therapy (to reposition "irritated" free-floating crystals in the semicircular canals) and surgical interruption of the posterior semicircular canal (to dampen response to angular head movement).

The presence or absence of auditory symptoms may also narrow the differential diagnosis for transient vertigo. **Ménière's disease, perilymphatic fistulas, and tumors of the glomus jugulare** all have auditory symptoms in addition to vertigo. Ménière's disease results from expansion of the endolymphatic compartment of the inner ear (often secondary to syphilis or head trauma) and presents with episodic vertigo (duration of 1-8 hours), low frequency sensorineural hearing loss, tinnitus (low tone and "blowing" in nature), and aural pressure. Both medical and surgical treatments focus on reducing endolymphatic pressure. Tumors of the glomus jugulare (a rare primary middle ear neoplasm) present with pulsatile tinnitus and hearing loss; unlike Ménière's disease, large glomus jugulare tumors may result in multiple neuropathies of the cranial nerves. The vertigo common to perilymphatic fistulas lasts only for a few seconds and often follows trauma sustained by the middle ear or erosion of the inner ear by a neoplasm or cholesteatoma. **Vestibular neuronitis** does not present with auditory impairment. A single attack of vertigo that may persist for days to weeks characterizes this disease; the etiology is unclear and treatment is symptomatic.

Tierney, 38th ed., pp 224-28.

52

(Block 2: Item 2)

(C)

Low-grade fever, arthralgias, and a rash of 3 days' duration hint at a viral prodrome. Suddenly, the patient has symptoms and signs (shortness of breath, tachypnea, tachycardia) of an acute anemia. The patient's hemoglobin has precipitously dropped from 32% (normal baseline for sickle cell patient) to 21%. **Measurement of a reticulocyte count** would be useful in differentiating between an aplastic anemia (low retic count—bone marrow suppressed) and an acute hemolytic anemia or vaso-occlusive crisis (high retic count—bone marrow responds appropriately). Parvovirus B19 can cause a severe aplastic anemia in sickle cell patients by destroying erythroid precursor cells in the marrow. Normal hosts with B19 disease usually present with erythema infectiosum (children) and/or arthropathy (usually, adults) with no significant decline in hematocrit. Immunosuppressed patients or patients with a chronic hemolytic anemia (e.g., sickle cell disease) cannot tolerate this 7-10 day shutoff of erythropoiesis and develop a severe transient aplastic crisis. The B19 virus infects and lyses erythroid precursors in the bone marrow; thus, these patients have a severe reticulocytopenia lasting 7-10 days. This patient will probably require erythrocyte transfusions and should be isolated to prevent nosocomial spread of the disease (patients with transient aplastic crisis, unlike their normal counterparts, are viremic).

Patients with sickle cell disease are homozygous for hemoglobin S, a protein with diminished solubility in the deoxy state. A gelatinous network of hemoglobin S distorts the erythrocyte membrane and makes it difficult or impossible for the rigid, "sticky" RBCs to flow through small blood vessels. Vaso-occlusive crises from trapping of sickled erythrocytes in end organ capillaries cause splenic ("autosplenectomy"), brain, eye, lung, marrow, and renal infarcts, aseptic necrosis of bone (osteomyelitis secondary to staphylococci or salmonellae), ankle ulcers, priapism, and "acute chest syndrome" (fever, chest pain and pulmonary infiltrates). Sickle cell patients almost always have chronic anemia and associated fatigue, pallor, decreased exercise tolerance, and when chronic, jaundice and gallstone (pigment stones) formation. There are three distinct types of acute episodes or "crises" – (1) Infarctive or painful crises: intense skeletal pain for days to weeks, fever, no change in hemoglobin, (2) Sequestration crises: acute pooling of RBCs in the spleen, sudden decrease in hemoglobin, usually in infants and children, and (3) Anemic (either aplastic or hemolytic) crises: uncommon, fall in hemoglobin, jaundice, may last hours to days. Acute vaso-occlusive events may be precipitated by infection, dehydration, or hypoxia. Management of patients with sickle cell disease includes avoidance of complications and treatment of crises. Folic acid (1 mg/day) and vaccinations against *Haemophilus influenzae* Type b, pneumococcus, and meningococcus. Some patients may also receive chronic transfusions to decrease crisis frequencies; this may lead to iron overload over time. Painful crises are usually treated with hydration, keeping the patient warm, and continuous infusional morphine for analgesia. Acute chest syndrome usually merits broad-spectrum antibiotics and, often, RBC or exchange-RBC transfusion. Controlled trials have demonstrated that hydroxyurea significantly reduces the rate of complications in sickle cell disease; hydroxyurea increases hemoglobin F levels by stimulating erythropoiesis in more primitive erythroid precursors and thereby reduces sickling. Severe cases (e.g., patients with a long history of transfusions or strokes) may benefit from allogenic bone marrow transplantation.

Fauci, 14th ed., pp 648-49, 1096-98.
Tierney, 38th ed., pp 497-99.

53

(Block 2: Item 3)

(E)

The differential diagnosis for an adolescent male with sudden onset of scrotal pain, inguinal tenderness, and scrotal absence of the ipsilateral testis should always include torsion of the testis and torsion of the testicular appendix or epididymis. This is a surgical emergency! **Immediate operation** to restore blood supply to the affected testis and prevent testicular infarction is mandatory. If facilities are available, color flow Doppler ultrasound of the testicle or nuclear scan can be done. However, this should not delay surgical exploration when the clinical suspicion for torsion is high. Complete torsion of the spermatic cord may result in testicular infarction within 4-6 hours. Classically, torsion of the testis occurs in the 10- to 20-year age group and presents with sudden onset of scrotal and lower abdominal pain and scrotal swelling. The exquisitely painful testis may have a "high lie" in relation to the other testis, and may even lie in the inguinal canal itself. The absence of voiding symptoms and a normal urinalysis also distinguish testicular torsion from epididymitis.

Tierney, 38th ed., pp 896-97.
Way, 10th ed., pp 968-69.

54

(Block 2: Item 4)

(A)

The differential diagnosis for a young, sexually active woman with abdominal pain includes gastrointestinal, genitourinary and reproductive disease—a long list! Guarding and tenderness to palpation in the right lower quadrant, absent bowel sounds, anorexia, nausea, low-grade fever, and a normal pelvic exam suggests **appendicitis**. At an early stage, appendicitis classically presents with diffuse abdominal pain, nausea (with or without vomiting), and anorexia. Within hours the pain localizes to the right lower quadrant (typically, over McBurney's point [one-third of the distance between the anterior superior iliac spine and the umbilicus]). The patient may have absent bowel sounds, rebound tenderness, guarding, a low-grade fever, and moderate leukocytosis (average WBC count is 15,000/mm^3) with neutrophilia. The psoas sign (pain on passive extension of the right hip) and the obturator sign (pain with passive flexion and internal rotation of the right hip) strongly suggest inflammation associated with appendicitis. Classic appendicitis merits no further studies, but imaging studies may be especially useful in young women (20 to 40 age group) who have the highest incidence of false-positive diagnosis (30-40%). Abdominal or transvaginal ultrasound has a diagnostic accuracy rate of 85%. An abdominal CT should be obtained to rule out periappendiceal abscess if appendiceal perforation is suspected. The treatment for uncomplicated appendicitis is surgical appendectomy, either via a laparotomy or by laparoscopic techniques. Preoperative antibiotics have also been shown to reduce postoperative wound infections.

Lack of sudden severe abdominal pain with diffuse abdominopelvic tenderness and shock places **ectopic pregnancy** lower on the differential; a pregnancy test and pelvic ultrasound are diagnostic. **Ovarian cysts** usually result in a disruption of hormonal cycles causing menstrual irregularities; a twisted ovarian cyst may cause sudden severe pain and would be tender to palpation on exam. **Tubo-ovarian abscesses** or acute salpingitis are associated with high fever, bilateral abdominal or pelvic tenderness, recent onset of menses, IUD use, and cervical motion tenderness. It is unlikely that this patient has a **ureteral calculus** since this condition presents with severe ureterorenal colic (abrupt costovertebral pain radiating to the ipsilateral lower abdominal quadrant), gross hematuria, nausea, vomiting, ileus, and urinary frequency and urgency (when the stone approaches the bladder).

Tierney, 38th ed., pp 608-09, 719.
Way, 10th ed., pp 610-11, 937.

55

(Block 2: Item 5)

(D)

Worsening peripheral edema, ascites, and hypertension in a previously healthy young woman suggests renal pathology. Elevated BUN and creatinine coupled with hypoalbuminemia and proteinuria are consequences of a reduced glomerular filtration rate (GFR) and a leaky glomerular basement membrane. These findings point to **glomerular renal disease.** Hypoalbuminemia causes a decrease in serum oncotic pressure and leads to peripheral edema, ascites, and pulmonary edema (basilar crackles). Hypertension is due to volume overload rather than activation of the renin-angiotensin axis (angiotensin II levels are typically low).

Interstitial renal disease also results in a reduction in GFR and increased BUN and creatinine; however, interstitial and tubular damage would generate sloughed cellular debris and casts, easily recognized in the urinalysis. In a majority of cases, **acute tubular necrosis** (ATN: acute renal failure due to tubular damage) is caused by ischemia (secondary to prerenal azotemia) and toxin exposure (antimicrobials, contrast media, cyclosporin, heavy metals, rhabdomyolysis, transfusion reactions, hemolytic anemias, multiple myeloma, etc.). The urinalysis in ATN appears muddy brown and may show pigmented casts, "muddy brown" casts, and epithelial cells and cell casts.

Congestive heart failure (CHF) and **cirrhosis of the liver** are both unlikely diagnoses given the lack of risk factors and classic physical findings associated with these diseases. Cirrhosis does result in hypoalbuminemia and decreased BUN from reduced synthetic capacity of the failing liver. Abnormalities on cardiac exam (e.g., S_3 or S_4), jugular venous distension, and marked pulmonary edema (with paroxysmal nocturnal dyspnea and orthopnea) are classic features of CHF.

Tierney, 38th ed., pp 869-71, 880-90.

56

(Block 2: Item 6)

(B)

Lapses in consciousness and a depressed gag reflex often predispose patients with seizure disorders to aspiration pneumonia. Bacteria from oropharyngeal and gastric secretions are transmitted to the lower airways, and an **anaerobic pneumonia** may then develop in the affected pulmonary segment or lobe. Bacteria responsible for aspiration pneumonia often colonize dependent lung zones (the posterior segments of the upper lobes and the superior and basilar segments of the lower lobes). The right lung has a higher incidence of aspiration pneumonia due to decreased angle between the right mainstem bronchus and the trachea. The onset of symptoms may be insidious, but most patients have a high fever, weight loss, malaise, and a cough with classic foul-smelling sputum at presentation. This nasty smelling sputum usually indicates a mixed bag of anaerobic bugs, commonly, *Prevotella melaninogenica*, anaerobic streptococci, *Bacteroides* species and *Fusobacterium nucleatum*. Aspiration pneumonia may progress to necrotizing pneumonia, lung abscess, or empyema. Treatment with clindamycin or β-lactam/β-lactamase inhibitor should be continued until the chest radiograph stabilizes.

Gram-positive and Gram-negative pneumonias do not produce foul-smelling sputum. The patient who aspirates in the hospital may have "mixed" aspiration pneumonia with enteric Gram-negative rods joining the anaerobes. Pneumonia secondary to ***Mycoplasma pneumoniae*** often presents with a more insidious course, a nonproductive cough, and diffuse patchy infiltrates on chest radiograph. A type of **chemical pneumonitis** (so-called Mendelson's syndrome) may result from the regurgitation and aspiration of gastric juices. This causes pulmonary inflammation and transudation of fluid into the alveolar space. This syndrome, in contrast to aspiration pneumonia, develops within hours, and the patient may become tachypneic, hypoxic and febrile. Sputum production is minimal and the chest radiograph can show complete "whiteout" within 8-24 hours.

Fauci, 14th ed., p 994.
Tierney, 38th ed., pp 289-90.

57

(Block 2: Item 7)

(F)

Thrombotic thrombocytopenic purpura (TTP) is disease of unknown etiology characterized by arteriolar lesions in end organs containing platelets and fibrin. The hallmarks of the disease are a microangiopathic hemolytic anemia, thrombocytopenia, markedly elevated LDH (lactate dehydrogenase), and normal coagulation studies. Neurologic and renal abnormalities (often only seen when the platelet count dips below 20,000-30,000/μL) and noninfectious fever contribute to the clinical picture of TTP. Taken together, these features are almost pathognomonic for TTP. TTP occurs in young adults between the ages of 20 and 50, with slightly more women affected than men. High estrogen levels (e.g., oral contraceptive use or pregnancy) can occasionally precipitate TTP; it is also encountered in the setting of HIV disease, SLE, scleroderma, and Sjogren's syndrome.

Confusion, headache, aphasia, and variability in the level of consciousness typify the waxing and waning neurologic features of TTP. The patient is often febrile without evidence of an infection and may appear acutely ill. As the patient in this question demonstrates, physical exam reveals petechiae (small non-blanchable erythematous lesions caused by thrombocytopenia), jaundice/icterus (secondary to the hemolytic anemia), and tachycardia (secondary to anemia). Patients may also develop pallor and purpura as well as abdominal pain/tenderness due to pancreatitis.

The severity of the anemia in TTP usually mirrors the trend of thrombocytopenia. Notably, fragmented red blood cells (schistocytes, helmet cells, triangle forms) are seen on the peripheral smear, consistent with a microangiopathic hemolytic anemia. Hemolysis also increases indirect bilirubin, and the LDH is markedly elevated in proportion to the severity of the hemolysis. A direct Coombs test is negative. White cells may also show an increase in band forms. Coagulation studies (prothrombin time, partial thromboplastin time, fibrinogen) are normal; sometimes infarcted tissue may initiate secondary disseminated intravascular coagulation (DIC). Fibrin split products may appear in acutely ill patients. Renal failure and an abnormal urinalysis may contribute to the constellation of laboratory findings.

Although TTP once heralded a dismal prognosis, prompt treatment with large-volume plasmaphoresis now results in a greater than 90% survival rate. Patients may need plasmaphoresis with plasma replacement once or twice daily. A rise in the platelet count and fall in the plasma LDH and a reduction in fragmented red cells measure response. Once patients begin responding, the frequency of plasmaphoresis can be reduced but may need to be continued for one to two months. Some patients also receive glucocorticoids and platelet-active agents (dipyridamole, aspirin, sulfinpyrazone); platelet transfusions should be avoided because they can initiate thrombotic events.

In addition to TTP, other causes of microangiopathic hemolytic anemia include hemolytic-uremic syndrome (HUS), DIC, prosthetic valve hemolysis, metastatic adenocarcinoma, malignant hypertension, and vasculitis. HUS is part of a spectrum of disease with TTP signified by neurologic compromise & severe thrombocytopenia and with HUS characterized by more significant renal failure. HUS is almost exclusively seen in children.

TTP is distinguished from **DIC** by normal coagulation studies and the absence of fibrin split products. **Idiopathic (autoimmune) thrombocytopenic purpura** (ITP) features isolated thrombocytopenia; unlike TTP, other hematopoietic cell lines are normal in ITP. **Meningococcal meningitis** can also present with petechiae, neurologic abnormalities, and thrombocytopenia; distinguishing features include positive Kerning and Brudzinski's signs as well as back and neck rigidity. DIC is a feared complication of meningococcal meningitis. Purulent spinal fluid with Gram-negative diplococci and positive cultures of CSF, blood, or petechial aspirates confirm the diagnosis. Autoimmune diseases such as **systemic lupus erythematosus (SLE)** may present with a hemolytic anemia (Coombs positive), mild thrombocytopenia, renal disease (proteinuria), and neurologic disease (seizures, psychosis). SLE patients present with joint symptoms, discoid rash, malar rash, photosensitivity, oral ulcers, and serositis; labs often reveal a positive antinuclear antibody (ANA) test and other immunologic abnormalities. Although both TTP and **sarcoidosis** affect multiple organ systems, sarcoidosis often presents with leukopenia, eosinophilia, hypercalcemia, and elevated erythrocyte sedimentation rate, none of which are characteristically seen in TTP. Sarcoidosis is a diagnosis by exclusion; definitive diagnosis requires histologic demonstration of noncaseating granulomas in biopsy specimens.

Fauci, 14th ed., pp 668-69.
Tierney, 38th ed., pp 308-09, 520-23, 812-15, 1309-10.

58

(Block 2: Item 8)

(B)

This young woman is likely dependent on oxycodone for chronic pain; abrupt cessation can cause **opiate withdrawal.** Diaphoresis, tachycardia, mydriasis, anxiety, flank discomfort, and insomnia are all features of opiate withdrawal. Withdrawal from severe opioid addiction can include diarrhea, weight loss, hemoconcentration, vomiting, spontaneous ejaculation and orgasm.

Tricyclic intoxication would result in higher serum concentration of amitriptyline; a serum amitriptyline level of 150 mg/dL is at the low end of the therapeutic range (150-250 mg/dL). Tricyclic intoxication would also resemble **anticholinergic poisoning**—tachycardia, mydriasis, dry mouth, flushed skin, muscle twitching, and decreased peristalsis—and quinidine-like cardiotoxic effects, most notably QRS interval widening. **Serotonin syndrome** can be precipitated when multiple medications that alter serotonin metabolism (classically, monoamine oxidase inhibitors and another serotonin reuptake inhibitor); the syndrome is characterized by rigidity, autonomic instability, myoclonus, confusion, hyperthermia, delirium and eventually coma. Although the patient complains of flank pain, a **renal calculus** is more commonly associated with sudden, severe colicky pain that may be accompanied by nausea, vomiting and microscopic hematuria (>5 rbc/hpf).

Murphy, 1st ed., pp 67.
Tierney, 38th ed., pp 1037-38, 1517-18, 1526.

59

(Block 2: Item 9)

(E)

Attention Deficit/Hyperactivity Disorder (ADHD) is a psychiatric condition that affects an estimated 3-5% of school-age children. Most of the children with ADHD are boys (sex ratios range from 4-9:1 [boys : girls]). Impulsivity, inattention, distractibility, and persistent overactivity typify the disease. DSM-IV criteria for ADHD mandate that the child exhibit inattentive or hyperactive symptoms before 7 years of age; the symptoms must also be present in at least two different settings (e.g., both home and school). The brief history presented for the 10-year-old boy appears to fit these criteria. That said, one should be careful to differentiate ADHD from age-appropriate behavior in active children, oppositional-defiant disorder, conduct disorder and other mood/anxiety disorders. Treatment of ADHD involves both pharmacotherapy and behavior modification. **Methylphenidate**, a psychostimulant, is the drug of first choice. Psychiatrists try to use the smallest effective dose and limit use to periods of greatest need due to long term side effects (weight loss and inhibited body growth).

Imipramine and **amitriptyline** are both tricyclic antidepressants (TCAs) with undesirable side effects including orthostatic hypotension, anticholinergic side effects, cardiac toxicity, and sexual dysfunction. Imipramine can be used for depression, chronic pain, panic, anxiety, and enuresis (bed-wetting). **Fluoxetine** is a selective serotonin reuptake inhibitor (SSRI) used most commonly for depression and also for treatment of panic attacks, bulimia, and obsessive compulsive disorder. **Haloperidol** is an antipsychotic used for childhood schizophrenia and for Tourette's syndrome.

Murphy, 1st ed., pp 34-35.

60

(Block 2: Item 10)

(I)

Bleeding (often gastrointestinal) commonly causes **iron deficiency** anemia in adults. A 54-year-old man with positive stool occult blood, a 20-lb. weight loss, an enlarged liver, and anemia (males: hematocrit < 41%, hemoglobin < 13.5 g/dL) should be evaluated for a colon/rectal neoplasm. Iron deficiency starts with depletion of total-body iron stores and a concomitant decrease in the serum ferritin (< 30 μg/L is a highly reliable indicator of iron deficiency). With low or absent iron stores, serum total iron-binding capacity (TIBC) rises. The mean corpuscular volume (MCV) of the red blood cells subsequently falls (< 85 fL) and the peripheral blood smear shows hypochromic, microcytic cells. Clinical symptoms include easy fatigability and tachypnea and palpitations on exertion. If the patient's iron deficiency is severe and prolonged, skin and mucosal changes (smooth tongue, brittle nails, cheilosis) and dysphagia (Plummer-Vinson syndrome: formation of esophageal webs) may occur.

Acute blood loss would likely present with orthostatic changes (a drop in blood pressure and tachycardia upon standing from a supine position). Constitutional symptoms such as weight loss and weakness may be seen in **acute myelogenous leukemia (AML), chronic lymphocytic leukemia (CLL), and chronic myelogenous leukemia (CML).** CML usually features a markedly elevated blood count (150,000/μL mean WBC at diagnosis) with a left-shifted myeloid series; the patient typically has mild to moderate anemia with normal RBC. Many patients are diagnosed with CLL after an incidental lymphocytosis is discovered; over half of patients have lymphadenopathy and hepatosplenomegaly (hepatomegaly in the absence of splenomegaly is extremely rare in CLL). The hallmark of acute leukemia is a combination a pancytopenia with circulating blasts (with granules [Auer rods] in AML); patients with AML usually have fever, fatigue, and may have bleeding in the skin and mucosal surfaces. **Folic acid deficiency** and ***Diphyllobothrium latum*** **infection**, a fish tapeworm causing vitamin B_{12} deficiency, would both present with megaloblastic anemia (MCV > 125); the peripheral smear features macro-ovalocytes and hypersegmented neutrophils. **Erythrocyte enzyme deficiency** (e.g., G6PD deficiency, pyruvate kinase deficiency) causes episodic hemolytic anemia; during periods of hemolysis, a reticulocytosis, increased serum indirect bilirubin, and "bite cells" on peripheral smear are commonly seen. The MCV is usually normal or increased in hemolytic anemia. **Hemochromatosis** results in increased accumulation of iron in the form of hemosiderin in the liver, heart, pancreas, adrenals, gonads, and kidneys; the clinical picture may feature hepatomegaly and hepatic insufficiency, arthropathy, skin pigmentation (bronze), diabetes mellitus, heart failure, and impotence. Finally, patients with **β-thalassemia trait** (β-thalassemia minor) have mild to moderate anemia with hematocrit between 32% and 38%. In comparison to iron deficiency anemia, patients with beta thalassemia trait have a more significant microcytosis (MCV ~ 55-75 fL), a more normal red blood cell count, no abnormalities in iron studies and a peripheral smear that appears more abnormal compared to the degree of anemia (hypochromia, microcytosis, target cells, basophilic stippling).

Fauci, 14th ed., pp 639-43.
Tierney, 38th ed., pp 485-513.

61

(Block 2: Item 11)

(C)

This patient's clinical presentation is most consistent with **influenza**. She has a normal chest X-ray, which would make pneumococcal, *H. influenzae*, or TB pneumonia unlikely. Patients with pertussis usually have low grade fevers, coryza, and conjunctivitis, followed by a prolonged period (6 weeks or more) of paroxysms of coughing and wheezing. Influenza, an orthomyxovirus, causes a common viral infection presenting with acute onset of chills, fever (lasting up to a week), myalgias, sore throat, headache, coryza, and a nonproductive cough. Transmission usually occurs via aerosolized droplet nuclei causing epidemics during the fall and winter months. Lab findings include leukopenia and occasionally proteinuria. Complications include secondary bacterial infection due to necrosis of the respiratory epithelium. Related acute sinusitis, otitis media, purulent bronchitis and pneumonia can be particularly problematic in the elderly. A trivalent influenza virus vaccine is engineered yearly to combat the most prevalent strains of influenza. The vaccine provides partial immunity for up to a year; adequate immunity is achieved about two weeks post vaccination. It is recommended yearly for people over 65 years, nursing home residents, patients with chronic lung, heart, metabolic or renal disease, hemoglobinopathies, or on immunosuppressive drugs, health care workers, and children and teenagers on chronic aspirin therapy (Reye's syndrome: rare and severe complication of influenza associated with aspirin use). Amantadine or rimantadine have been shown to reduce the attack rate in naïve individuals exposed to influenza; these antivirals must be started immediately and continued for 10 days.

The **Hemophilus influenzae Type b ("Hib") vaccine** is recommended for all children and for adults who have sickle cell disease, are asplenic, transplant recipients, and those receiving certain types of chemotherapy. The **pneumococcal vaccine** contains polysaccharides from the capsule of the 23 most common strains of *Streptococcus pneumoniae*. It is recommended for healthy adults over 65 years old, those without a spleen, persons with sickle cell disease, chronic cardiopulmonary disease (e.g., COPD), cirrhosis, alcoholics, and the immunocompromised. A single dose usually results in life-long immunity, but revaccination every 6 years should be considered in asplenic and other high-risk patients (remember that the spleen is the key defense against encapsulated organisms such as *Streptococcus pneumoniae*, *Hemophilus influenzae*, and *Neisseria meningitidis*). Vaccination against **pertussis** is not recommended in adults. The whole-cell pertussis component of the DTP vaccine for children may elicit adverse reactions in adults. **BCG vaccine** is a live, attenuated strain of *M. bovis*, used for the prevention of tuberculosis. BCG is currently only considered for tuberculin-negative individuals who are repeatedly in contact with persons with untreated or ineffectively treated TB and who cannot receive isoniazid chemoprophylaxis. It is not recommended for routine use in the U.S.

Tierney, 38th ed., pp 296, 1217-21, 1279-81.

62

(Block 2: Item 12)

(D)

Pseudotumor cerebri or idiopathic intracranial hypertension usually occurs in young obese women who present with bifrontal headaches, diplopia, and other visual disturbances secondary to papilledema and abducens nerve (CN VI) dysfunction. Papilledema is optic disk swelling due to increased intracranial pressure (ICP). Proper evaluation of papilledema necessitates head CT or MR imaging to rule out an intracranial mass. If the radiologic data are normal, it is important to complete a lumbar puncture to assess opening pressures, characteristically elevated in pseudotumor cerebri. The sum of these findings points to pseudotumor cerebri, a diagnosis of exclusion. Treatment with acetazolamide reduces the amount of CSF production; aggressive weight loss is also important but often unsuccessful. If these interventions fail, visual field loss may progress and lumboperitoneal shunting or optic nerve sheath fenestrations may be required to prevent blindness.

Migraines are classically lateralized to one side of the head and usually occur in episodes that build in intensity over several hours. In many cases, they do not conform to any one pattern. Migraines can be associated with nausea, vomiting, anorexia, photophobia, phonophobia, and diplopia. Visual disturbances and hallucinations as well as focal disturbances (numbness, aphasia) may occur. **Tension headaches** are often described as generalized pressure-like pain (like having your head in a vice); they do not present with any focal neurologic findings. Papilledema is not a feature of migraine or tension headaches. Papillitis (swelling of the optic disk) can be seen in **optic neuritis**. Optic neuritis is defined by a sudden, unilateral loss of acuity and color vision, pain with eye movements, scotomas, and afferent pupillary light defect. Optic neuritis may proceed to optic atrophy if destruction of the optic nerve has occurred. This disease is commonly associated with demyelinating diseases such as multiple sclerosis. **Posterior fossa tumors** (medulloblastomas, astrocytomas, pontine gliomas) account for 60% of pediatric CNS tumors. Symptoms and signs of increased ICP due to a brain neoplasm can include vomiting, headache (worse upon awakening), papilledema, mental dysfunction, personality changes, and abducens nerve palsy. Suspicion of a CNS tumor merits appropriate imaging studies.

Fauci, 14th ed., p 167.
Tierney, 38th ed., pp 203-04, 932-33, 958.
Way, 10th ed., pp 841-42.

63

(Block 2: Item 13)

(C)

Fat embolism is a dreaded complication of long bone (e.g., femur) fractures. Although immobilization after surgery is a risk factor for deep venous thrombosis and secondary pulmonary thromboembolism (PE), fat embolization more closely fits this clinical scenario. Regardless of the etiology, PE may cause dyspnea, tachycardia, and low grade fever. Tachypnea, distended neck veins, and accentuated pulmonic component of S_2 are also found in PE. Fat emboli can also lodge in the cerebral vasculature and result in confusion. An important cutaneous sign of fat emboli are petechiae; they typically appear on the upper body 2 to 3 days after a major injury.

Adverse drug reactions (analgesics) are an unlikely explanation for this presentation. For example, NSAIDs can cause hypertension, interstitial nephritis, gastrointestinal ulceration and hemorrhage, renal dysfunction and, rarely, anaphylaxis. Patients with **disseminated intravascular coagulation** (DIC) may bleed from venipuncture sites, nasal mucosa, gums, and the gastrointestinal tract; thrombosis may be manifest by digital ischemia and gangrene. DIC is usually caused by a serious illness—sepsis, severe tissue injury, obstetric complications, cancer, and major transfusion reactions. Patients in **hypovolemic** shock usually have tachycardia followed by low systemic blood pressure, altered mental status, oliguria, and metabolic acidosis. **Thrombocytopenia** can cause bleeding into the skin or mucosa (purpura, petechiae) and would not alone account for the severity of this patient's signs and symptoms.

Fauci, 14th ed., pp 326, 427-29, 1469.
Tierney, 38th ed., pp 19, 481, 532.

64

(Block 2: Item 14)

(C)

An otherwise asymptomatic teenage boy with multiple episodes of syncope during exercise and a family history significant for sudden death at a young age is highly suspicious for cardiogenic syncope. Historical points favoring a cardiac source of syncope include: sudden onset without warning and lack of aura or seizure activity or sensation of rapid heartbeat prior to loss of consciousness. In addition to the history and physical exam, an **ECG** may narrow the differential between mechanical problems, disorders of automaticity, conduction disorders, and tachyarrhythmias. This picture seems most consistent with hypertrophic obstructive cardiomyopathy (HCM, also known as idiopathic hypertrophic subaortic stenosis), given that the syncope occurred with exercise and the strong family history of sudden death. HCM stems from hypertrophy of the myocardium (sometimes involving the intraventricular septum disproportionately) that narrows the left ventricular outflow tract during systole. Syncope in HCM occurs when cardiac output decreases due to increased outflow obstruction; factors that increase myocardial contractility (such as exercise) or decrease diastolic LV filling worsen the condition. Some variants of HCM show an autosomal dominant mode of inheritance; the prognosis is related to the specific gene mutation. HCM may also present with dyspnea and chest pain; patients usually come to medical attention in early adulthood. Cardiac exam may reveal a sustained apical impulse, S_4, or a systolic ejection murmur. Because LV hypertrophy is almost universal, an **ECG** would add weight to a diagnosis of HCM. The ECG may also show septal Q-waves without any evidence of a myocardial infarction. Echocardiography is diagnostic. Beta-blockers, calcium channel blockers, excision of part of the septum, and implantable defibrillators have all been used in the treatment of HCM.

Seizures may also present with syncope, and an **electroencephalogram** (EEG) may be diagnostic. Often patients with a seizure disorder may note prodromal symptoms (headache, mood alterations, lethargy, myoclonic jerking) or an aura; a postictal headache and confusion is also common. Patients may also have syncopal episodes secondary to an intrinsic neurologic disorder such as an intracranial mass or transient ischemic attacks. It would be rare to present with syncope alone and no other neurological signs or symptoms; these diagnoses may be pursued with a **CT scan of the head** or MR imaging. If an intracranial process is suspected, **lumbar puncture** should not be performed because fatal herniation can result. Finally, neurocardiogenic syncope is a common cause of syncope that can be tested on a **tilt table test**. Sudden positional change causes syncope secondary to overcompensation in vasovagal tone.

Tierney, 38th ed., pp 402, 416-17, 938-39.

65

(Block 2: Item 15)

(A)

This patient's clinical picture is most consistent with subacute infectious endocarditis (IE). Dental procedures often cause transient bacteremia; patients with preexisting valvular disease (as well as intravenous drug users and the immunocompromised) are susceptible to developing infective endocarditis. Like most patients with IE, this man has persistent fever and malaise, tachycardia, neutrophilia with bandemia, and hematuria. Subacute IE may also feature anemia of chronic disease, a normal WBC, and an elevated erythrocyte sedimentation rate (ESR). Ninety percent of patients with IE have either new or changing heart murmurs (right-sided infections sometimes have no murmur). Embolization or immunologically-related events may also cause cough, dyspnea, arthralgias or arthritis, diarrhea, abdominal pain, petechiae, "splinter" hemorrhages, Osler nodes, Janeway lesions, Roth spots, pallor, and splenomegaly.

One of the major criteria for the diagnosis of IE includes a positive blood culture for a bacteria that typically causes IE from two separate blood cultures. *Streptococcus viridans*, a **Gram-positive cocci in chains**, causes 90% of all native valve endocarditis in non-intravenous drug users.

Other Gram-positive bacteria that can cause native valve endocarditis include *Staphylococcus aureus* (20% of all cases; **Gram-positive cocci in clusters**) and *Enterococcus faecalis* (5-10% of all cases; **Gram-positive cocci in short chains**). Only a small percentage of native valve endocarditis is due to **Gram-negative organisms** or fungi.

Tierney, 38th ed., pp 1303-08.

66

(Block 2: Item 16)

(E)

Systemic lupus erythematosus (SLE) is an inflammatory autoimmune disease that occurs mainly in young (reproductive-age) women and may have multiple system involvement. The clinical manifestations that define SLE are, in large part, due to lodging of antigen-antibody complexes in capillaries of end organs or to autoantibody destruction of "self" cells. The clinical course of SLE can wax and wane; likewise, the severity of SLE spans a wide spectrum. This patient meets 6 of the criteria for SLE (4 out of the 11 criteria required for diagnosis): oral ulcers, arthritis, renal disease (3+ proteinuria), thrombocytopenia, and lymphopenia (<1500/μL), a false-positive serologic test for syphilis (RPR), and a positive antinuclear antibody. Prominent in this patient are joint symptoms, with or without active synovitis, that occur in many SLE patients and may be an early manifestation of the disease. X-rays rarely show erosive changes. Anti-native DNA antibodies correlate with disease activity; generalized inflammation accounts for an elevated erythrocyte sedimentation rate. Urinalysis may contain sediment (RBCs and WBCs, with or without casts) and proteinuria, indicative of renal lesions.

Although this patient is sexually active and has severe arthralgia, **disseminated gonococcal disease** is less likely because it features migratory polyarthritis and a characteristic skin rash consisting of small necrotic pustules over the extremities (palms and soles). Also, it is unlikely that the young woman has **polyarticular arthritis** since this commonly affects 5 or more joints. She does not have the clinical tetrad of **Reiter's syndrome**—urethritis, conjunctivitis, mucocutaneous lesions and arthritis. Finally, although the patient does have a nonpainful oral ulcer and a positive RPR, she does not have any of the other symptoms of **secondary syphilis**—maculopapular skin rash, weeping papules, nontender lymphadenopathy, or meningitis, hepatitis, osteitis, and iritis.

Tierney, 38th ed., pp 774, 812-14, 829-30, 1337.

67

(Block 2: Item 17)

(B)

In order to diagnose hyperthyroidism, it is important to **measure serum thyroid-stimulating hormone** (TSH) levels. TSH is suppressed in primary hyperthyroidism; free T_4 and T_3 levels are increased. This patient exhibits many of the signs and symptoms of primary hyperthyroidism (thyrotoxicosis)—tachycardia, palpitations (exacerbated by caffeine intake), stare and lid lag, flow murmur, and a diffusely enlarged, firm thyroid gland (goiter).

In the absence of other cardiac findings or symptoms, there is no urgency to pursue a full cardiac workup including **ambulatory ECG monitoring, echocardiography** or **MUGA scan** (multiple-gated radionuclide cardiac scan used for evaluating myocardial infarction) in the setting of thyrotoxicosis. Patients with pheochromocytomas present with "attacks" of headache, perspiration, and palpitation and not with stare, lid lag, and an enlarged thyroid; 95% of patients with pheochromocytoma have hypertension. Lab findings include normal serum T_4 and TSH and **elevated urine catecholamines**.

Tierney, 38th ed., pp 1074-80.

68

(Block 2: Item 18)

(A)

Perineal pain is a common complication of episiotomies. Second-degree lacerations extend into the perineal body but do not involve the anal sphincter. Tylenol with codeine or Darvocet are often sufficient analgesia after vaginal births. An anesthetic spray (such as Americaine) may help with episiotomy pain as well as **sitz baths**. A sitz bath is a warm water bath taken in the sitting position that covers only the hips and buttocks and may contain medication. Some obstetricians prefer ice-water sitz baths for the first 24 hours after delivery.

Without evidence of episiotomy infection, hematoma or breakdown, there is no reason to begin **intravenous ampicillin** therapy. **Local injection of lidocaine into the perineum** is usually performed immediately prior to the episiotomy repair. **Epidural analgesia** might be effective for labor pain (although it can have possible adverse effects). It would not be realistic after delivery.

Benson, 2nd ed., p 86.
Callahan, 1st ed., pp 29-30.

69

(Block 2: Item 19)

(B)

In a case where both a patient (who is minor) and his parents decline experimental therapy, the most appropriate course of action is to **discharge the child routinely**. This decision preserves the patient's autonomy. The experimental therapy holds uncertain benefit for the child and may even do harm. Thus, there are no issues of malevolence or medical neglect if the treatment is withheld from the child. There is no reason to **petition the court for an order for the experimental treatment** against the wishes of the child and his parents, **report the parents to child protective services** for medical neglect, nor **discharge the child against medical advice**.

Tierney, 38th ed., pp 106-07.

70

(Block 2: Item 20)

(C)

Hyperthyroidism is a hypermetabolic state manifest as nervousness, restlessness, heat intolerance, increased sweating, fatigue, increased bowel motility, weight loss, and cardiac irregularities. One of the hallmarks of hyperthyroidism is increased free T_3 and T_4 and suppressed levels of TSH.

Attention-deficit/hyperactivity disorder (ADHD) may feature irritability, distractibility, restlessness and failing school performance. DSM-IV criteria for ADHD mandate that the child exhibit inattentive or hyperactive symptoms before 7 years of age. Although some patients with **diabetes mellitus** may present with irritability and weight loss, they characteristically have polyuria, thirst, polyphagia, recurrent blurred vision, vulvovaginitis or pruritus, peripheral neuropathy, and nocturnal enuresis. **Pituitary adenomas** *very* rarely hypersecrete TSH causing thyrotoxicosis. Regardless of the hormone that they secrete or if they are nonfunctional, the most common deficiencies found with pituitary adenomas are (in descending order) growth hormone, gonadal hormones, ACTH and, rarely, thyroid. Hyperprolactinemia, due to pituitary stalk compression, is also a very common manifestation of adenomas; women may have amenorrhea, galactorrhea, and breast tenderness, and men may present with decreased libido and breast enlargement or tenderness. Patients with pituitary adenomas may have visual symptoms (bilateral hemianopsia) and/or headaches due to anatomical changes within the sella. Pediatric patients with **thyroid cancer** often have normal thyroid function tests, painless swelling of the thyroid gland, and a past history of irradiation to the head or neck.

Tierney, 38th ed., pp 1051-52, 1075-76, 1122.

71

(Block 2: Item 21)

(D)

Sarcoptes scabiei is a human mite and causes one of the most common pruritic dermatoses. Patients with scabies almost always complain of severe itching; the presence of "runs" of multiple erythematous papules on skin creases such as finger webs, wrist creases, and the heels of the palm is classic. The infestation may occur around the nipples in females and on the penile shaft and glans in males; typically, the disease spares the head and neck. The disease is usually acquired by close contact (e.g., sharing bedding) with an infested individual. Diagnosis is confirmed by microscopic demonstration of the mite, ova or brown dots of feces. Treatment must involve all infected groups; bedding and clothing must be laundered or set aside for two weeks. A topical cream such as 1% lindane or 5% permethrin is applied for 8-12 hours and may be repeated in one week.

Measles and **varicella viruses** can also cause pruritus and characteristic rashes. The measles virus causes an irregular, brick-red maculopapular rash that begins on the face and trunk, progresses to involve the extremities and finally appears on the palms and soles. The rash appears 3-4 days after a prodrome of fever, coryza, conjunctivitis, and cough. Varicella is also typified by a prodrome of fever and malaise. The varicella rash is papular at first, then vesicular, pustular, and crusting. All stages may be present simultaneously and the distribution of lesions is centripetal. The **Epstein-Barr virus** often affects young people between the ages of 10-35 and can result in a maculopapular rash resembling rubella; EBV also causes fever, sore throat, lymphadenopathy and splenomegaly in patients. **Group A streptococcus** causes skin infections after contact with another infected individual or after a preceding streptococcal respiratory infection. Impetigo is a vesicular, pustular lesion with a honey, crusted, "stuck-on" appearance. Erysipelas, another skin infection caused by group A streptococci, is a superficial cellulitis, often on the face. It can be painful and is well demarcated from surrounding skin. Group A streptococcus may also be the culprit in cellulitis and lymphangitis.

Tierney, 38th ed., pp 165, 1260, 1265, 1292.

72

(Block 2: Item 22)

(E)

Acute pancreatitis is characterized by deep epigastric pain radiating to the back associated with nausea, vomiting, weakness, and abdominal tenderness and distention. Consistent with acute pancreatitis, the patient's lab values reveal a leukocytosis and elevation in serum amylase. His hematocrit is elevated, suggesting hemoconcentration due to dehydration. There is also a history of alcohol abuse. Treatment requires pain management (meperidine, 100-150 mg every 3-4 hours as needed), intravenous hydration, nasogastric decompression (for abdominal distention and vomiting) and withholding of food and liquids by mouth until the patient is pain free and has bowel sounds. This patient needs to be **admitted to the hospital for the above medical management**.

IV antibiotics should not be used prophylactically in the setting of acute pancreatitis; their use is indicated if the patient has septicemia, pancreatic abscess, or necrotic pancreatitis. **Surgical therapy** is indicated for excision and drainage of foci of pancreatic necrosis; for gallstone pancreatitis, cholecystectomy is performed after the acute pancreatitis subsides. **Endoscopy** may be performed to rule out associated gastrointestinal bleeding due to alcoholic gastritis, bleeding varices, stress ulceration, or to remove bile duct stones in those with severe gallstone pancreatitis (ERCP, endoscopic retrograde cholangiopancreatography).

Ferri, 3rd ed., pp 351-52.
Tierney, 38th ed., pp 671-74.

73

(Block 2: Item 23)

(C)

Hyperandrogenic insulin-resistant acanthosis nigricans syndrome, also referred to as the "HAIR-AN syndrome," describes clinical features associated with this uncommon disease. Between 1-5% of hyperandrogenic women suffer from this disorder. It is characterized by extremely high circulating levels of insulin (generally > 80 μU/mL in the fasting state and > 300 μU/mL following an oral glucose tolerance test). The high levels of circulating insulin are generally due to an insulin receptor and/or a post-receptor defect. Rarely these women have circulating anti-insulin antibodies. Acanthosis nigricans is an associated dermatologic condition manifest as hyperpigmented, velvety, thickened skin lesions on the neck or other skin fold areas, and is highly correlated with the degree of insulin resistance in HAIR-AN patients. Girls with HAIR-AN syndrome are usually severely hyperandrogenic, and can even be masculinized. Polycystic ovaries are a feature of HAIR-AN, resulting in excess production of the androgens androstenedione and testosterone. Excess androstenedione is converted to estrone (a precursor of estrogen) and results in increased total estrogen. High estrogen causes suppression of pituitary FSH, a relative increase in LH (increased LH:FSH ratio), and increased production of prolactin. Constant LH stimulation of the ovary results in anovulation, cysts, and theca cell hyperplasia with concomitant increases in androgen synthesis. Elevated LH levels may also stimulate excessive adrenal androgen production (increased dehydroepiandrosterone sulfate, DHEAS). Clinical features of androgen excess include hirsutism, amenorrhea, virilization, and obesity.

In evaluating a previously healthy sexually active woman presenting with new onset secondary amenorrhea and recent weight gain, **pregnancy** should always be considered. Normal pregnancy results in elevation of ACTH and plasma cortisol, which is responsible for some of the "pseudo-Cushingoid" features of pregnancy such as hyperpigmentation, striae gravidarum, and impaired glucose tolerance. Androgens (in particular, DHEAS and testosterone) are produced by the fetal adrenal cortex and fetal testis in response to the elevation of ACTH and HCG, respectively. This may cause mild hirsutism during pregnancy. However, enlarged ovaries, an increased LH:FSH ratio, and/or a prior history of abnormal menses would not normally be associated with pregnancy. **Addison's disease** (primary adrenocortical deficiency) is relatively rare and presents with symptoms of gradual adrenal cortical destruction—weight loss, GI distress, anorexia, hypotension, and increased pigmentation. The increased pigmentation may be noticeable in exposed areas or mucous membranes and is caused by increased MSH (melanocyte stimulating hormone) activity, secondary to increased ACTH in response to cortisol deficiency. Laboratory values would show subnormal levels of cortisol and aldosterone, which would fail to increase after ACTH administration. However, glucose would tend to be normal to low, and DHEA-S, testosterone, and prolactin would all be expected to be normal. **21-hydroxylase deficiency** is the most common enzyme deficient state associated with congenital adrenal hyperplasia. This disorder is an autosomal recessive trait often diagnosed in adolescent women after puberty, who present with severe hirsutism or virilism while having normal menses. 21-hydroxylase converts 17-hydroxyprogesterone to deoxycortisol and, in its absence, results in an accumulation of 17-hydroxyprogesterone and its metabolites androstenedione and testosterone. The most common ovarian neoplasm is the **benign cystic teratoma** (dermoid cyst) that is not known to have any endocrinological effects. Other tumors such as granulosa-theca cell tumors may produce excessive androgens or estrogen and thus inhibit menstruation.

Bennet, 4th ed., pp 515.
Hacker, 2nd ed., pp 53-55, 69, 344, 362, 537.
Speroff, 5th ed., pp 463-70.

74

(Block 2: Item 24)

(E)

The most common malignancy in young men is testicular cancer; the average age at diagnosis is 32 years. Malignancy needs to be considered in any patient that presents with a nontender testicular mass or swelling. **Tumors** of the testis are usually painless, firm, solid lesions within the substance of the testis. Masses within the testis are usually malignant and those from the epididymis and spermatic cord structures are usually benign. Transillumination differentiates solid from cystic lesions; tumors do not transilluminate.

Epididymitis is a usually painful inflammation of the epididymis and, in sexually active young men, most often caused by *Chlamydia trachomatis* or *Neisseria gonorrhoeae*. Infection with the organisms is commonly associated with an asymptomatic or subclinical urethritis (70% of cases). Gram stain of the urethral discharge is usually purulent and shows greater than 5 neutrophils per high power field or Gram-negative diplococci within neutrophils (*Neisseria).* Epididymitis in patients over 35 years may present with unilateral testicular pain, swelling, tenderness, and fever, but this usually occurs following instrumentation or surgery. A **hematoma** from blunt trauma might initially present with local pain, discoloration, swelling, and tenderness. They usually regress on their own, or enlarge, sometimes requiring surgical intervention. A hematoma would not likely present as a discrete, unchanging, nontender mass. A **hernia** extending into the scrotum (termed a complete [indirect] inguinal hernia) occurs when a loop of bowel or intra-abdominal tissue is allowed passage through the internal inguinal ring and the inguinal canal into the scrotum. A common history would describe an intermittently present mass that may or may not be painful, and/or associated with strenuous activity. On physical exam, the mass may be tender, feel or sound like bowel, and be reducible with gentle pressure. A **hydrocele** is a cystic accumulation of clear serous fluid within the tunica vaginalis and, in adults, may be the result of epididymo-orchitis or trauma. It may also be seen in association with a large inguinal hernia, which can obstruct normal venous and lymphatic drainage, and thus create a hydrocele. An identifying characteristic of a hydrocele is that it transilluminates. 10% of testicular tumors have an associated hydrocele.

Jarell, 2nd ed., pp 45-46, 408.
Tierney, 38th ed., p 896.

75

(Block 2: Item 25)

(D)

Leiomyomas (fibroids) are common benign smooth muscle tumors; 20% of women develop them by 40 years of age. They are estrogen dependent and therefore usually occur during the reproductive years. Leiomyomas may enlarge during pregnancy or with oral contraception use. Fibroids lack a cellular capsule and consequently undergo degenerative changes as they enlarge. **Pedunculated submucous leiomyomas** may project through the cervix and may present as "beefy red tissue" in the os. Most leiomyomas are asymptomatic, but metrorrhagia (heavy periods) and intense pain may sometimes occur. This is a result of submucous myomas ulcerating through the endometrial lining or of carneous (red) degeneration within a fibroid caused by interstitial hemorrhage from vascular occlusion.

Carcinoma of the cervix is usually detected at an early stage by routine Pap smear and may be asymptomatic. In invasive cervical cancer, vaginal discharge and abnormal bleeding are the most common symptoms. Other symptoms such as pelvic pain or visible lesions (to the naked eye) are indicative of advanced disease, and would likely have systemic manifestations as well. The most common symptom of **endometrial cancer** is post-menopausal bleeding. In the premenopausal patient, menorrhagia or intermenstrual bleeding may be the presenting symptom. On examination, an expanded cervix or cervical os may indicate extension of the disease from the corpus to the cervix, and would again suggest advanced disease, not likely to be associated with acute labor-like pains. If a patient has had a menses within the last month, then it is unlikely that this scenario represents an **incomplete abortion**. **Sarcoma of the uterus** is relatively rare and tends to be quite advanced at the time of diagnosis.

Hacker, 2nd ed., pp 348-50, 577-78, 583, 592.

76

(Block 2: Item 26)

(E)

Patients with emphysema are prone to acute COPD exacerbations that manifest as worsening dyspnea, fatigue, and, ultimately, respiratory failure. Initial attempts to improve oxygenation in COPD patients with an acute exacerbation include low flow oxygen (**24-35% oxygen by Venturi mask** is preferred to **1-3 L/min via nasal cannula**). Inhaled β_2-adrenergic agonists **(bronchodilators)** such as metaproterenol, terbutaline, or albuterol are also used in the treatment of acute COPD exacerbations. Adequate oxygenation must be maintained, even in the face of increasing hypercapnia; thus, **discontinuation of the oxygen** is not a viable option.

This patient, however, is suffering from severe CO_2 retention (the ABG [6 L/min O_2] reveals a $PaCO_2$ of 95 mm Hg!). Hypercapnic respiratory failure occurs with acute CO_2 retention (Pa CO_2 > 45-55 mm Hg) and the development of respiratory acidosis (pH < 7.35). High flow oxygen therapy in a patient with COPD may cause hypercapnia by suppressing respiratory drive. The most important decision in this patient is whether or not to **intubate**. The decision to begin **mechanical ventilation** is a clinical judgement that takes into account the reversibility of the underlying disease as well as the patient's general medical condition. For example, a patient with COPD may "live" normally at $PaCO_2$ > 60 mm Hg and have a respiratory rate > 30/min; ABG values alone should not dictate the ultimate need for mechanical ventilation. However, in addition to severe hypercapnia and acidemia, this 60-year-old man has a 3-day history of respiratory decline (dyspnea, cough, sputum) and is now lethargic, incoherent and confused (impaired consciousness is a typical sign of hypercapnia). Clinical assessment and ABG values make endotracheal intubation and mechanical ventilation the best option for this patient.

Ferri, 3rd ed., p 601.
Tierney, 38th ed., pp 275, 334.

77

(Block 2: Item 27)

(A)

This scenario is consistent with a case of erysipelas; a break in the skin allows bacteria to invade and rapidly spread via the skin lymphatics. Erysipelas has an acute onset, spreads rapidly, and can lead to bacteremia and death if not treated with antibiotics (intravenous penicillin or 1st generation cephalosporin therapy) in a timely manner. Erysipelas is a superficial form of cellulitis, frequently involves the face or cheek, and is caused by **beta-hemolytic streptococci (group A)**. Erysipelas manifests as an edematous, erythematous, painful lesion with an elevated advancing margin, which may vesiculate and form surface bullae. Symptoms of erysipelas include pain, malaise, chills, fever, and progressive swelling that may cause the eyelids to be swollen shut. Lab tests may show a leukocytosis, an increased sedimentation rate, and positive blood cultures.

Haemophilus influenzae Type b is associated with pneumonia, epiglottitis, and, rarely, meningitis; the Hib vaccine is now a routine childhood immunization. ***Streptococcus pneumoniae*** is the most common cause of community-acquired pneumonia and meningitis in adults (especially in alcoholics). ***Neisseria meningitidis*** is the culprit for purulent meningitis and meningococcemia. **Herpes simplex virus** primarily affects the oral or genital areas and is characterized by recurrent outbreaks of small grouped vesicles on an erythematous base, often following a trigger such as stress, illness, trauma, or sun exposure.

Tierney, 38th ed., pp 140, 154-55, 1129, 1173, 1292, 1310.

78

(Block 2: Item 28)

(C)

Sarcoidosis is a systemic disease of unknown etiology characterized by noncaseating granulomas involving the lung, skin, eyes, spleen, liver, kidney and heart (in order of frequency of involvement). The incidence is highest in African American women and Caucasians of Northern European descent. Initial symptoms include malaise, fever, and progressive dyspnea; skin rashes, erythema nodosum, hepato-splenomegaly, lymphadenopathy and arthralgia may also be present. Onset of the disease is usually in the fourth and fifth decades. Bilateral hilar lymphadenopathy or lung involvement is present on chest X-ray in 90% of sarcoid cases. Radiographic findings determine staging and consequently affect prognosis. Hilar lymphadenopathy alone is classified as Stage I and carries the best prognosis, followed by lymph-adenopathy plus parenchymal involvement (Stage II), and finally parenchymal involvement alone (Stage III), which is most likely to progress to chronic pulmonary fibrosis. Lymph nodes are involved in almost all cases, specifically the hilar and mediastinal nodes. Skin lesions are seen in one-third to one-half of cases and may appear as subcutaneous nodules, elevated, erythematous plaques, or flat, scaly lesions similar to those of lupus erythematosus. Spleen and liver involvement is even less common (fewer than 20% of cases). Histologically, involved tissues show **noncaseating granulomas** composed of epithelioid cells with Langhans' and foreign body-type giant cells. Other characteristic microscopic features are asteroid bodies (stellate inclusions within giant cells) and Schaumann bodies (laminated concretions composed of calcium and proteins).

Reed Sternberg cells are distinctive neoplastic giant cells ("owl's eyes") that are pathognomonic for Hodgkin's disease (HD) and induce the accumulation of reactive lymphocytes, histiocytes and granulocytes. Hodgkin's disease is characterized by painless lymphadenopathy (often a painless neck mass) and "B" symptoms (low-grade fever, weight loss, night sweats). **Fat-laden or "foamy" histiocytes** may be found in the lymph nodes and skin lesions of patients with lepromatous leprosy. A **paravascular homogenous eosinophilic infiltrate** may be seen in allergic granulomatosis and angiitis (the Churg-Strauss syndrome); the pathological features are very similar to polyarteritis nodosa, but this syndrome is characterized by bronchial asthma, eosinophilia, and granulomas involving pulmonary and splenic vessels, peripheral nerves, and skin. **Vasculitis with giant cells** is often seen in giant cell (temporal) arteritis (granulomatous inflammation of the aorta and its major branches with a predilection for the extracranial branches of the carotid artery) and Takayasu's arteritis ("pulseless disease"). Wegner's granulomatosis also features perivascular inflammation with giant cells in the lungs and upper airways.

Cotran, 6th ed., pp 370, 385-86, 490-97, 648, 670-74, 734-35, 738.

79

(Block 2: Item 29)

(B)

Diverticular disease of the colon is most prevalent in patients over 60 years; a fiber-poor diet is thought to be a risk factor. Diverticula are produced by herniation of the mucosa and submucosa through the colonic muscle wall, usually near mesenteric vessels. They are variable in size and number, and, although most are asymptomatic, common presentations include lower GI bleeding and diverticulitis. **Acute diverticulitis** usually presents as left lower quadrant (LLQ) abdominal pain, low-grade fever, and leukocytosis. Often, symptoms are mild enough to delay patients from seeking medical attention for several days. Diverticulitis may recur and lead to complications such as perforation, obstruction, stricture, and/or fistulas (bladder, bowel, and uterus), which may necessitate operative intervention. Nonoperative treatment consists of bowel rest (NPO) with or without nasogastric suction, IV fluids, and antibiotics (metronidazole plus ciprofloxacin or trimethoprim-sulfamethoxazole). Localized abscesses can be identified and drained using CT guidance.

Acute appendicitis classically occurs in patients 10 to 30 years of age, and begins with vague, periumbilical or epigastric pain that then shifts to the right lower quadrant (RLQ). Anorexia, nausea, vomiting, low-grade fever, and leukocytosis are prominent features. Typically, symptoms progress rapidly and require emergent appendectomy. **Acute pyelonephritis** usually develops from an ascending lower urinary tract infection and is characterized by flank pain (CVA tenderness), fever, chills, and irritative voiding symptoms (urgency, frequency, and dysuria). Nausea, vomiting, and diarrhea are also common symptoms. Lab findings may include leukocytosis with a left shift; urinalysis would likely show pyuria, bacteruria, hematuria, and/or WBC casts. Although GI disorders such as diverticulitis or appendicitis are usually associated with a normal urinalysis, adjacent inflammation may result in pyuria and/or hematuria on urinalysis. **Acute cholecystitis** is usually caused by obstruction due to gallstones and characteristically produces pain in the right upper quadrant (RUQ) or epigastric region. Symptoms may be precipitated by a large or fatty meal and include severe, steady pain in the RUQ, nausea and vomiting, and fever and leukocytosis. Lab findings may reveal abnormal elevations in bilirubin, aminotransferase (AST), and alkaline phosphatase. **Spontaneous bacterial peritonitis** (SBP) occurs in patients with preexisting chronic liver disease and ascites. Ascitic fluid becomes infected in the absence of an intra-abdominal source of infection (versus infection from an intra-abdominal source, which is termed secondary bacterial peritonitis). Cirrhotic patients with low ascitic fluid protein are especially prone to develop SBP. The most common symptoms of SBP are fever and diffuse abdominal pain. Paracentesis and lab testing of ascitic fluid (cell count, cultures, protein, LDH, glucose, gram stain) can help make a definitive diagnosis.

Tierney, 38th ed., pp 560-61, 608-09, 665-66, 901.

80

(Block 2: Item 30)

(E)

Hirsutism is excessive hair growth in androgen-sensitive areas of the body such as face, chest, pubic area, and ears. Mild, isolated hirsutism is often a result of a familial tendency and generally is not associated with adrenal or ovarian dysfunction. Idiopathic or familial hirsutism may be due to a slight increase in androstanediol glucuronide, a metabolite of dihydrotestosterone produced by the skin. These patients do not present with signs of defeminization or virilization such as amenorrhea, clitoromegaly, deepening of the voice, or frontal balding. Evaluation of hirsutism is especially important when signs of androgen excess (virilization and menstrual dysfunction) are present, since androgen-producing tumors (Sertoli-Leydig tumors, granulosa-theca cell tumors, dysgerminomas, and hilar cell tumors) must be considered as a possible cause. One of the most common causes of hirsutism (50% of cases of clinical hirsutism) is polycystic ovarian syndrome (PCOS). These patients characteristically present with enlarged ovaries, obesity, and amenorrhea. Androgen overproduction (by the ovaries) is stimulated by elevated plasma LH (luteinizing hormone) (LH:FSH > 2.0). Adult-onset hirsutism has also been linked, in about 2% of patients, to a partial defect in adrenal 21-hydroxylase; these patients do not have salt wasting. Exogenous drugs (phenytoin, minoxidil, diazoxide, and cyclosporin) should be considered as a possible cause of hirsutism. Rare causes of hirsutism include adrenal carcinoma, ACTH-induced Cushing's syndrome, acromegaly, and ovarian luteoma of pregnancy.

Diagnostic evaluation should begin with a measurement of **serum testosterone** and **dehydroepiandrosterone sulfate** (DHEA-S). Serum androgen evaluation screens for rare occult adrenal or ovarian neoplasms. If the testosterone is over 200 ng/dL an ovarian ultrasound is used to look for a functioning ovarian tumor. If DHEA-S is over 700 mcgm/dL, an MRI is ordered to rule out an adrenal tumor. If the DHEA-S is between 500 - 700 mcgm/dL, then further endocrine testing is needed to rule out adrenal hyperfunction such as hyperplasia.

FSH and **LH** levels should be measured if amenorrhea due to ovarian failure or PCOS is a concern. If the woman is anovulatory, she also should have **prolactin, T4** and TSH levels checked. A breast exam should be done to check for galactorrhea. If the woman has long-standing anovulation, an endometrial biopsy may be indicated. Evaluation of "late-onset" 21-hydroxylase deficiency (late-onset congenital adrenal hyperplasia) requires measurement of **17α-hydroxyprogesterone**. Prolactin and **17α-hydroxyprogesterone** may also be ordered if: the excess hair growth has been present since puberty, there is a strong family history of hirsutism, ethnic background is Ashkenazi Jewish, a woman is found to be shorter than other family members or there is evidence of defeminization such as a decrease in breast size. These risk factors can be associated with genetic causes of adrenal hirsutism that do not always result in elevated DHEA-S levels. Acromegaly, caused by GH (growth hormone)-secreting pituitary tumors, can demonstrate elevations in serum prolactin, either by direct secretion or by pressure on the pituitary stalk. ACTH-induced Cushing's syndrome (truncal obesity, purple striae, amenorrhea, hypertension, osteoporosis, glucosuria, and hirsutism) would reveal abnormally high 24-hour urine free cortisol (after a dexamethasone suppression test) and/or elevated **serum cortisol** levels at baseline. Measurement of **estrogen** and **progesterone** may be elevated in conditions (such as ACTH-induced Cushing's syndrome) that increase all of the steroid hormones.

Bennet, 4th ed., pp 514-17.
Tierney, 38th ed., pp 1097-1100.

81

(Block 2: Item 31)

(C)

Orbital cellulitis usually occurs in children and is characterized by the acute onset of fever, unilateral periorbital pain, proptosis, restriction of extraocular movement, and swelling and erythema of the lids. The most common route of orbital infection is from the adjacent paranasal sinuses, but may also occur through direct inoculation following penetrating trauma to the eye or skin. Orbital cellulitis requires immediate treatment with IV antibiotics to prevent optic nerve damage and spread of the infection.

Since on examination the disc margins are sharp and no retinal abnormalities are found, it is probable that the infection has not spread to the cavernous sinus. Symptoms of **cavernous sinus thrombosis** include decreased visual acuity, afferent pupillary reflex defect, color vision deficit, visual field defect, diminished pupillary reflexes, and papilledema. **Lateral sinus thrombosis** (LST) is an intracranial complication of otitis media. Classic symptoms of LST include a "picket fence" fever pattern, chills, progressive anemia (especially with β-hemolytic Strep), headache, and papilledema. **Periorbital cellulitis** is an acute infection of the tissues surrounding the eye, including the fat pads behind the eyeball. Unlike orbital cellulitis that actually involves the orbit, periorbital cellulitis does not cause proptosis or limit movements of the eye, because the infection is limited to that part of the orbital cavity anterior to the orbital septum. However, periorbital cellulitis may progress to orbital cellulitis if left untreated. **Sagittal sinus thrombosis** impairs venous drainage of the brain, which may result in focal or diffuse cerebral edema and cortical venous infarcts that are often hemorrhagic. Presentation may include nonspecific symptoms such as headache, seizures, and nausea, as well as focal neurologic complaints. This diagnosis is often clinically overlooked.

Gorbach, 2nd ed., pp 1373-76.

82

(Block 2: Item 32)

(A)

Herpes genitalis (human herpes virus Type 2) is one of the most common sexually transmitted diseases (30% of women test positive for HSV 2 antibody). It is most often acquired through unprotected sexual intercourse, and the incubation period lasts 2 to 7 days. The infection presents as small patches of painful, ulcerating vesicles involving the vulvar, vaginal, or ectocervical surfaces. Urinary symptoms such as urinary retention or dysuria may develop along with bilateral inguinal adenopathy, fever and malaise. Lesions may persist for 2 to 6 weeks, and recurrence is likely to occur. Herpes genitalis is treated with oral and/or topical **acyclovir**, which, although not curative, has been shown to reduce the frequency and severity of initial and future outbreaks.

Ganciclovir is a nucleotide analog that competitively inhibits viral DNA polymerase by decreasing the rate of chain elongation. It acts through the same mechanism as acyclovir, but unlike acyclovir is effective against CMV (cytomegalovirus) infection. **Immune globulin** can be used for Hepatitis A and B prevention and for preventing infection in patients who are severely immunocompromised with observed immunoglobulin deficiencies (CLL, multiple myeloma, post bone marrow transplantation patients). **Interferons** block virus replication, stimulate natural killer (NK) cells, and activate tumoricidal macrophages; they are used in the treatment of leukemia and various tumors. **Zidovidine (AZT)** blocks viral replication through selective incorporation into viral DNA by reverse transcriptase and is used in the treatment of HIV infection.

DeCherney, 8th ed., pp 703-05.
Mycek, 2nd ed., pp 365-66, 368-69, 397-98.
Tierney, 38th ed., p 100.

83

(Block 2: Item 33)

(A)

Indomethacin is a particularly potent NSAID and is often used for inflammatory conditions involving the joints such as rheumatoid arthritis, acute gout, ankylosing spondylitis. Indomethacin's anti-inflammatory effects stem from inhibition of prostaglandin synthesis through selective blockade of cyclooxygenase. Unfortunately, toxicity (usually dose-related) limits its use; chronic administration of indomethacin and its use in patients in whom renal vasodilation is prostaglandin-dependent are especially concerning. In the elderly population, because of reduced effective circulating volume in conditions such as congestive heart failure (CHF), cirrhosis, dehydration, and chronic renal disease, prerenal azotemia may result from indomethacin use. In addition, NSAIDS are known to precipitate acute interstitial nephritis and renal insufficiency in some patients. Signs of renal failure include pedal edema, oliguria, and an increase in creatinine and BUN (blood urea nitrogen). Since indomethacin is known to cause renal toxicity, in a previously healthy patient, the first step would be to **discontinue indomethacin**. Renal insufficiency usually resolves upon discontinuation of the offending agent.

If symptoms do not resolve and creatinine and BUN do not return to baseline, then further evaluation will be indicated. Urinalysis and **measurement of urine sodium and creatinine** will be the next diagnostic tests to differentiate between prerenal and postrenal azotemia as well as intrinsic renal disease. If fluid overload is suspected, a **diuretic agent** might then be administered. If renal parenchymal diseases, obstruction, or chronic renal failure is suspected, **renal ultrasonography** provides a noninvasive, reliable method of evaluation. If the kidneys are normal-sized in a patient presenting with renal failure, a biopsy might be indicated to rule out amyloidosis or other intrinsic causes of renal disease.

Bennet, 4th ed., pp 237-38, 240.
Katzung, 7th ed., pp 588-89.

84

(Block 2: Item 34)

(A)

Chorioamnionitis (infection of the amniotic fluid surrounding the fetus) is correlated with preterm labor and prolonged rupture of membranes (ROM). It is the most common cause of neonatal sepsis and meningitis, which have a high rate of mortality (25% for term neonates and over 50% for preterm neonates). Maternal fever, maternal leukocytosis, uterine tenderness, and fetal tachycardia are hallmark signs of chorioamnionitis. Group B streptococcus (GBS) is one organism that causes chorioamnionitis; a significant proportion of the population is colonized with GBS in the vagina and the rectum. Broad-spectrum IV antibiotics should be started immediately; often, antibiotic prophylaxis is recommended in the settings of preterm delivery and prolonged ROM. **Ampicillin** and **gentamycin** are the standard first-line regimen for chorioamnionitis. Ampicillin has good aerobic Gram-negative coverage and also facilitates the synergistic effect of gentamycin, an aminoglycoside that covers organisms such as *E. coli*, streptococci (enterococcus) as well as *Pseudomonas* and *Proteus.*

Clindamycin is especially effective against anaerobes such as *Clostridium* and *Bacteroides* species. **Ciprofloxacin**, a quinolone, is active against a broad range of organisms (both Gram-positive and Gram-negative bacteria) with the exception of anaerobes. Although the combination of ciprofloxacin with clindamycin might provide coverage for a polymicrobial chorioamnionitis, they do not possess the potent synergism of ampicillin and gentamycin. **Erythromycin** is the treatment of choice for pneumonia, and is useful against Gram-positive cocci in penicillin-allergic patients. **Penicillin** also has better activity against Gram-positive organisms when compared to **ampicillin**, which is more effective against Gram-negative bacteria. **Metronidazole** is effective against anaerobes and protozoa.

Callahan, 1st ed., p 44.
DeCherney, 8th ed., pp 582-85.

85

(Block 2: Item 35)

(C)

When either survival or mortality is compared in two groups, it is essential that both groups have the same starting point (e.g., onset of symptoms, first diagnosis, or beginning of treatment). Discrepancies in starting points result in **"lead-time" bias**, whereby making an earlier diagnosis through screening prolongs the interval from diagnosis to death but does not necessarily change the date of death (i.e. prolong life). Lead-time bias in a cohort study implies that the screening group got diagnosed earlier than the unscreened group and knew of their disease for a longer time. Assessing mortality rates in the two groups rather than duration of the disease would be a more appropriate way to analyze these data.

Length-time bias occurs when screening preferentially detects cases with more slowly progressive disease. Since the randomized, controlled trial looked at survival rates rather than duration of illness, length-time bias should not be a problem. **Statistical power** is the probability that a study will detect a difference between groups if the difference really exists. If a statistically significant difference is found, then power is adequate. If no difference is found, then we have to wonder if there is truly no difference, or if the power was not adequate to demonstrate it. One of the major benefits of randomized clinical trials is that they minimize the distortive effects of **confounding**. Randomization is likely to distribute confounding variables equally among treatment and control groups, making these factors unlikely to affect the analysis. It is implausible that there was **misclassification of lung cancer** in the randomized, controlled study.

Friedman, 4th ed., pp 188-91, 198-201, 218-19, 328.

---

86 & 87

(Block 2: Items 36 & 37)

(A) & (E)

respectively

The most severe and acute transfusion reactions result from major antigen mismatches, specifically of the ABO system. Although these antigens are routinely tested prior to transfusion, **patient misidentification and mislabeling** sometimes results in hemolytic transfusion reactions that can be fatal. The incidence of a fatal hemolytic reaction is 1 in 100,000 units, and **ABO incompatibility** due to human error is the most common cause. During a hemolytic transfusion reaction, isoantibodies against A and/or B antigens activate complement and cause rapid intravascular lysis of incompatible red blood cells. This releases free hemoglobin into the plasma, and can result in hemoglobinuria (reddish-brown urine). Other symptoms of an acute hemolytic transfusion reaction include anxiety, nausea, flushing, pain at the infusion site, and chest or back pain. Lower back pain is a common complaint and thought to be due to ischemic muscle pain or vasospasm rather than kidney pain from developing renal failure. Nonspecific symptoms of shock and DIC (disseminated intravascular coagulation) such as fever and chills, dyspnea, hypotension, and tachycardia may also occur. The clinical severity of an ABO-incompatible blood transfusion is dependent on the degree of complement activation.

Other **minor antigens** such as the Rh, Jk (Kidd), Fy (Duffy) or Kell blood group systems can also produce hemolytic reactions, but are typically less severe, take place at a slower rate, and cause extravascular hemolysis. **Preformed antibodies to leukocyte antigens** can cause non-hemolytic febrile reactions, which are characterized by fever and shaking chills, and result from the release of cytokines (IL-1, IL-6, TNF-α) from macrophages, monocytes, granulocytes, or lymphocytes. Following several transfusions, patients may be sensitized by leukocyte antigens and develop febrile reactions to subsequent transfusions. The standard recommendation to prevent febrile reactions is to maintain a leukocyte level of less than 5×10^8 in transfused blood through washing, centrifugation, or filtration. **Erythrocyte washing** removes plasma and reduces leukocytes in order to prevent HLA alloimmunization, virus transmission, and febrile reactions. Bacterial contamination of blood can occur during venipuncture or component preparation. However, bacterial growth in refrigerated blood is uncommon and is usually limited to Gram-negative organisms that grow well at 4°C such as *Yersinia enterocolitica* or *Citrobacter* species. Transfusion of contaminated blood can result in septicemia and endotoxic shock with symptoms such as fever, flushing, cramps, DIC, renal failure, and cardiovascular collapse. However, this is distinguished from intravascular hemolytic reactions by the absence of hemoglobinemia and hemoglobinuria. **Adherence to sterile technique and preservation** can help prevent this complication. Lastly, intravenous catheter infections can cause bacteremia, and sepsis, which may present with similar symptoms. However, onset of symptoms would not be associated with the transfusion, and would appear more gradual and progressive. **Daily changing of peripheral IV sites** is a labor-intensive preventive measure against IV catheter infections.

Fauci, 13th ed., pp 1792-93.
Tierney, 38th ed., pp 535-36.

88

(Block 2: Item 38)

(F)

Symptoms of a typical panic attack include a sudden, overwhelming sense of fear accompanied by physical manifestations such as chest pain, shortness of breath, palpitations or tachycardia, trembling, sweating, nausea or GI distress, and numbness or tingling sensations (paresthesias). The intensity of anxiety usually peaks within 10 minutes and resolves in approximately 20-30 minutes. **Panic disorder** usually consists of unexpected, recurrent panic attacks and tends to be familial. Patients suffering from panic disorder are at risk for developing major depression and/or substance abuse. Abrupt cessation of alcohol or anxiolytics drugs may also precipitate a panic attack.

Alcohol withdrawal would present with some similar symptoms (tremor, tachycardia, tachypnea, generalized anxiety, and GI distress); however, symptoms would usually begin 5-10 hours after discontinuing alcohol intake, peak in intensity on day 2 to 3, and improve by day 4 or 5. Also, patients suffering from withdrawal would have prominent autonomic symptoms including tremulousness, tachycardia, and hypertension; they may also appear confused and ataxic, experience delirium tremens or seizures, and may show physical signs of chronic alcoholism. Patients diagnosed with

post-traumatic stress disorder (PTSD) have experienced a catastrophic event or severe trauma outside the range of normal human experience. They reexperience the trauma through recurrent dreams, distressing recollections of the event, or exposure to reminders of the traumatic event. Acutely, symptoms begin within six months of the trauma and last less than six months. Patients with PTSD show symptoms of increased arousal (insomnia, irritability, difficulty concentrating, hypervigilance, exaggerated startle response), persistent avoidance of stimuli associated with the trauma, and decreased general responsiveness (decreased interest, detachment, restricted affect). **Somatization disorder** is a chronic illness characterized by multiple, recurrent physical symptoms with no organic basis that begins before age thirty. A diagnosis of somatization disorder requires that symptoms occur outside the context of panic attacks, cause impaired social or occupational functioning, and result in medical treatment/attention being sought. Anxiety and depression are commonly associated symptoms. Although medical causes of anxiety should not be overlooked, with a normal physical examination, normal lab studies, an ECG without abnormalities, and no history of medical problems, it is unlikely that this patient has an organic basis for her anxiety.

Fauci, 13th ed., pp 2409-12.
Goldman, 4th ed., pp 284-86.

89

(Block 2: Item 39)

(C)

Hyperthyroidism ("thyrotoxicosis") is associated with increased levels of circulating thyroxine (free T4) and consequent suppression of TSH (thyroid stimulating hormone). Patients can present with a range of symptoms including nervousness, weight loss, increased sweating, fatigue, irritability, heat intolerance, loose stools, and menstrual irregularity. On physical examination, patients may have warm moist skin, fine resting tremors, tachycardia or atrial fibrillation, hyperreflexia, and a stare or lid lag. The most common form of hyperthyroidism is an autoimmune disorder called Graves' disease, in which autoantibodies bind to the TSH receptor, and stimulate hyperactivity of the thyroid cells. Graves' disease is more prevalent in women (8:1), and usually occurs between 20-40 years of age.

Symptoms of hyperthyroidism may overlap with those of a **pheochromocytoma**, which causes a similar hypermetabolic state (tachycardia, weight loss, sweating). Patients with pheochromocytomas describe longer, episodic histories of symptoms than patients with hyperthyroidism who tend to have histories of constant, daily symptoms after onset. They can be differentiated by laboratory tests such as urinary metanephrines and vanillylmandelic acid (VMA). The most common manifestation of a pheochromocytoma are "attacks" of headaches, palpitations, and perspiration; often patients present with a distinct hypertensive crisis or hypertension that responds poorly to standard antihypertensive therapy. Although sweating, anxiety, and tremulousness may be associated with **hypoglycemia**, these symptoms are usually acute and a result of neurogenic autonomic discharge. Typically patients present with CNS symptoms such as blurred vision, diplopia, headache, slurred speech, and weakness. The most common cause of hypoglycemia is iatrogenic in nature (due to insulin or hypoglycemic agents), although missing a meal or overzealous exercise may contribute to the situation. Neurogenic symptoms (tremor, sweating, and tachycardia) may be blunted in chronic hypoglycemia due to the body's adaptation to low glucose levels. Finally, because the patient's physical manifestations are suggestive of organic disease, it is unlikely that the patient's anxiety is psychiatric in nature. Also, in anxiety related to psychiatric disorders (panic disorder, PTSD), skin is usually cold and clammy, and weight loss is often accompanied by anorexia versus an increase in appetite associated with hyperthyroidism.

Tierney, 38th ed., pp 1074-76, 1155-60.

90

(Block 2: Item 40)

(D)

Lead is contained in a variety of compounds/products such as car batteries, paints, pottery, plumbing, and gasoline. Toxicity usually results from repeated exposure and is characterized by dysfunction of the gastrointestinal system, the hematopoietic system, and the central and peripheral nervous systems. Systemic manifestations include colicky abdominal pain, constipation, headache, gum discoloration, motor neuropathy (wrist or foot drop), and anemia. **Acute encephalopathy** is a sign of severe toxicity. Laboratory findings particularly suggestive of chronic lead poisoning are microcytic anemia with basophilic stippling and elevated free erythrocyte protoporphyrin. Patients with severe intoxication (encephalopathy or lead levels above 70-100 μg/dL) are treated with IV or IM edetate calcium disodium ($CaNa_2EDTA$) and possibly oral penicillamine or dimercaprol (BAL).

Wernicke's encephalopathy results from thiamine deficiency usually in the context of chronic alcoholism and produces an *acute* confusional state, ataxia and ophthalmoplegia (CN VI). A peripheral blood smear would be likely to show macrocytosis and symptoms would improve following treatment with thiamine. In **Huntington's disease**, onset of symptoms occurs at age 40 to 50 in individuals with a genetic predisposition (autosomal dominant gene), and is characterized by gradual, progressive dementia and movement disturbances (chorea, rigidity, akinesia). Huntington's is not associated with any hematologic abnormalities. **Diabetic**

polyneuropathy generally affects the distal lower limbs more than the upper limbs, but is usually symmetric. 70% of cases are mixed sensory, motor and autonomic, while the remaining 30% are primarily sensory. Common symptoms are numbness, pain, and paresthesias, but may also be associated with footdrop due to nerve compression and/or sensory loss. Impaired proprioception and vibratory sense is seen in **tabes dorsalis** (late stage neurosyphilis). An absent Achilles reflex is present in 94% of patients. Tabes dorsalis would present with other manifestations of tertiary syphilis such as Argyll-Robertson pupils (accommodate but react poorly to light), muscular hypotonia/hyporeflexia, wide-based gait, pain crises (gastric, laryngeal, urethral), neurogenic bladder and Charcot joints. **Parkinson's disease** is a chronic neurodegenerative disease distinguished by tremor, rigidity, bradykinesia, and postural instability; mild dementia may also occur.

Aminoff, 3rd ed., pp 19-20, 170-01, 197, 204-05, 224-25.

91

(Block 2: Item 41)

(F)

Multiple sclerosis (MS) is an incurable, progressive demyelinating disease, with a peak incidence between ages 20 to 40; women are more commonly affected than men. Common initial manifestations of disease are focal weakness, numbness, tingling or unsteadiness in a limb, diplopia, sudden loss or blurring of vision in one eye (optic neuritis), and bladder sphincter disturbances (urinary urgency or hesitancy). Symptoms are often episodic and may disappear leaving a residual deficit; they may reoccur months or years later along with new symptoms. Optic neuritis may begin as unilateral visual blurring and is associated with orbital pain, usually worsening with eye movement. On physical examination, patients may display a dilated pupil, decreased visual acuity, and a paracentral blind spot (scotoma). Internuclear ophthalmoplegia (INO) is also fairly common in MS and is marked by loss of adduction on horizontal gaze, nystagmus in the abducting eye, and preservation of convergence. Bilateral INO is virtually diagnostic of multiple sclerosis.

Wernicke's encephalopathy is a rare cause of internuclear ophthalmoplegia; however, confusion, ataxia, and chronic alcoholism that are major features of Wernicke's are not present in this patient. Lesions or tumors at the level of the pons **(pontine glioma)** may produce disturbances in horizontal conjugate gaze, but this consists of eye deviation toward the side of the hemiparesis. A **medulloblastoma** is a posterior fossa tumor that is common in children, but rare in adults. Patients commonly present with an occipital headache, vomiting, ataxia, hydrocephalus, and visual disturbances. **Lateral medullary syndrome** (also known as Wallenberg's syndrome) results from occlusion of the vertebral artery (or, less often, the posterior inferior cerebellar artery); common symptoms include pain, numbness, impaired sensation, ataxia, nystagmus, diplopia, Horner's syndrome (ptosis, myosis, anhydrosis), vertigo, and impaired pain, heat sensation, and paralysis/weakness of the contralateral extremities.

Aminoff, 3rd ed., pp 111, 142-44, 158-59.
Fauci, 13th ed., pp 2244, 2267, 2287-94.

92

(Block 2: Item 42)

(G)

A patient with a long history of smoking is at increased risk for developing **pneumonia** due to impaired mucociliary action, increased bronchial mucous secretion, and alveolar macrophage dysfunction. Cigarette smoke contains irritants, ciliotoxins, and carcinogens that compromise pulmonary function. Studies have also correlated cigarette smoking with respiratory infections (pneumonia, influenza), cancer, COPD (chronic obstructive pulmonary disease), and atherosclerotic cardiovascular disease. A patient with acute onset fever, cough productive of purulent sputum, shortness of breath, and pleuritic chest pain displays symptoms of a "typical" pneumonia, most likely caused by a community-acquired bacterial pathogens such as *Streptococcus pneumoniae.* Physical examination findings characteristic of pneumonia include rhonchi, rales (crackles), wheezes, and egophony ('e' to 'a' changes on lung auscultation), which are often found in areas of radiographic abnormalities (infiltrates). Although a smoking history carries with it a significant risk for cancer, a patient with a **primary lung carcinoma** or **metastatic disease** would probably present with anorexia or weight loss as well as chronic hemoptysis, dyspnea, hoarseness, and/or cough. On chest X-ray, carcinoma might show up as an enlarging mass, infiltrate, atelectasis, cavitation or pleural effusion (a lung neoplasm can obstruct a lobe and cause pneumonia). The presence of an infiltrate on chest X-ray makes **COPD, CHF, asthma**, and **bronchitis** less likely as primary diagnoses. No doubt that with an 80 pack-year history this patient may have underlying COPD.

Fauci, 13th ed., pp 1184-91, 2434-35.
Tierney, 38th ed., p 298.

93

(Block 2: Item 43)

(E)

Cystic fibrosis (CF) is an autosomal recessive trait caused by a single deletion in the cystic fibrosis transmembrane conductance regulator (CFTR) gene; this defect results in abnormal chloride and water transport across cell membranes. This causes abnormal mucus secretion (often thick and viscous), impaired mucociliary function, and exocrine gland dysfunction. In young adults and children, CF is the most common cause of chronic lung disease. Pulmonary manifestations include acute and chronic bronchitis, bronchiectasis, recurrent pneumonia, atelectasis, and peribronchial & parenchymal scarring. Common respiratory pathogens include *Staphylococcus aureus, Haemophilus influenzae* and *Pseudomonas aeruginosa* (which characteristically produces copious amounts of yellow-green sputum). Pancreatic insufficiency and consequent steatorrhea (fat malabsorption) as well as infertility are commonly associated features. On chest radiograph, hyperinflation, bronchiectasis, interstitial markings and nodular opacities are often present. A "sweat test" showing a sweat chloride concentration above 80 meq/L is diagnostic of CF in adults. Cystic fibrosis is treated with symptomatic and preventative measures such as chest physiotherapy, bronchodilators, vaccinations (pneumococcal and influenza), antibiotics, and inhaled DNase. Definitive treatment of CF consists of lung transplantation and, potentially, gene therapy; few CF patients live beyond 35 years. In healthy young adults, pneumonia tends to be acute, short lived, and resolve with antibiotics unless underlying lung disease or an immunocompromised state exists. Other causes of hemoptysis include lung cancer, pulmonary embolus, bronchiectasis, tuberculosis (TB), pulmonary edema, systemic lupus erythematosus (SLE), Goodpasture's syndrome, and Wegener's granulomatosis.

Tierney, 38th ed., pp 281-82.

94

(Block 2: Item 44)

(N)

Tuberculosis (TB) is transmitted from person to person via respiratory droplets and is caused by the aerobic organism *Mycobacterium tuberculosis.* During primary infection (usually asymptomatic), macrophages in the lung ingest the TB bacillus, multiply, and spread via the lymphatics and bloodstream. The body's immune system then responds by walling off mycobacteria by granulomatous inflammation. These lesions may undergo central caseous necrosis and appear as cavitating lesions on chest

X-ray. In the majority of cases, organisms remain dormant but viable for years until the host's defense mechanisms are compromised; reactivation of the disease then occurs (secondary tuberculosis). Reactivation lesions usually occur in the apices of the lungs whereas primary lesions are more often seen in the lower lobes. The risk of infection and disease is highest in immunocompromised patients (especially those with HIV), and immigrants from Southeast Asia, Africa, and Latin America, where there is a high incidence of tuberculosis. Pulmonary tuberculosis is characterized by fatigue, weight loss, anorexia, fever, night sweats, and cough. Symptoms often begin with a non-productive cough that later may become productive of purulent or blood-tinged sputum. On physical exam, signs of chronic weight loss may be present along with upper lobe rales (crackles) and/or rhonchi, which may be heard on auscultation. On chest X-ray, reactivation tuberculosis is associated with cavitary apical infiltrates, nodules, and pneumatic infiltrates.

Fungal **pneumonia** caused by an organism such as *Aspergillus* can produce cavitating lesions in the lung; however, this is usually seen in immunocompromised individuals with an underlying chronic disease. Pulmonary lesions would not be confined to the upper lobes, and fungus may also disseminate to other organs (liver, brain and spleen). Significant weight loss raises a red flag for cancer. However, **primary lung cancer** in nonsmokers is uncommon and initial symptoms would not generally include fever, which is more indicative of an infectious process. **Metastatic disease** is also unlikely without other symptoms, physical exam findings, or lab abnormalities. Also, initial metastasis would probably be more likely to seed the lower lungs (according to blood flow distribution) rather than the upper lobes.

Tierney, 38th ed., pp 291-93.

95

(Block 2: Item 45)

(G)

Although many women with *Trichomonas vaginalis* infection are asymptomatic, they classically present with labial pruritus (itching), vaginal discharge, or both. Dysuria and dyspareunia (pain during intercourse) from labial irritation, as well as bad odor, are also common complaints. Symptoms often occur during or immediately follow menstruation. The typical finding on pelvic exam is a copious, yellow-green, foul-smelling, frothy vaginal discharge. The cervix may be covered with discrete red patches ("strawberry cervix"). Under the microscope, saline preparation ("wet mount") of the discharge reveals a motile, flagellated protozoan. The sample must be viewed quickly; room temperature immobilizes the trichomonads, and they are difficult to identify unless they are wriggling around on the slide. **Metronidazole** (Flagyl) in a single 2 g oral dose, or 500 mg orally twice a day for one week, is the treatment of choice for trichomonal vaginitis. Since *T. vaginalis* is a sexually transmitted disease, sexual partners should be treated simultaneously, and the patient should be counseled and screened for other STDs.

The symptoms and signs of trichomonal vaginitis can be confused with those of bacterial vaginosis, also known as *Gardnerella* vaginitis. Classically, bacterial vaginosis results in a thin white discharge and patients are more likely to notice a foul odor. This syndrome is thought to be caused by changes in the vaginal bacterial flora including loss of *Lactobacilli*, which result in increased vaginal pH and proliferation of multiple aerobic and anaerobic bacteria. *Gardnerella vaginalis*, a small, non-motile, pleomorphic rod is a common pathogen found in vaginosis, and its presence is demonstrated on a wet mount by "clue cells"—vaginal epithelial cells covered with dark specks which represent bacteria. The characteristic "fishy" odor of bacterial vaginosis is caused by anaerobic bacteria such as *Bacteroides* and *Peptostreptococcus*, and is especially noticeable when potassium hydroxide is applied to the slide ("whiff test"). Like trichomonal vaginitis, the treatment of choice for bacterial vaginosis is **metronidazole** (oral or as a vaginal cream). This syndrome is not thought to be sexually transmitted, though some have advocated the treatment of sexual partners in recurring cases.

Benson, 1st ed., pp 36-37.
Dale, pp 13-14.

96

(Block 2: Item 46)

(H)

Candidal vaginitis, the common "yeast infection," is usually caused by overgrowth of endogenous *Candida* rather than by exogenous infection. Vaginal secretions of 25-50% of asymptomatic women yield small quantities of *Candida*. Risk factors for symptomatic candidal infection include diabetes, pregnancy, HIV infection, and use of broad-spectrum antibiotics or corticosteroids. The most common symptoms are pruritus, a thick, white, "curdlike" discharge, vulvar erythema, and occasionally dyspareunia. Onset of candidal vaginitis is often prior to the menstruation. Wet mount preparation with 10% potassium hydroxide slide reveals pseudohyphae (filaments) and spores. Effective topical antifungal treatments include **miconazole, clotrimazole, butoconazole, tioconazole, terconazole, and nystatin**. A single dose of **oral fluconazole** is also effective.

Griseofulvin is an antifungal medication that inhibits the growth of some dermatophytes (in humans, these include Trichophyton, Microsporum, and Epidermophyton). It has an affinity for skin and keratin, and is thereby ideal for hair and nail infections. Griseofulvin can thus be used to treat tinea capitis, tinea corporis and tinea unguium (nail infection, also called onychomycosis). Oral itraconazole is now the treatment of choice for onychomycosis. **Acyclovir** is an antiviral medication used in the treatment of varicella and herpes simplex (HSV) infections. HSV infection is characterized by tingling or itching preceding vesicular eruptions in small patches that erode into painful ulcers. Varicella is characterized by vesicles that rupture and crust over. **Ceftriaxone** is the drug of choice for treatment of uncomplicated gonorrhea, which presents with purulent vaginal discharge, frequency and dysuria. It is often given with doxycycline or **tetracycline** to treat Chlamydia, since these STDs commonly occur simultaneously. Chlamydia can cause similar symptoms, though it is frequently asymptomatic. **Erythromycin** is useful as a substitute for tetracyclines in the treatment of Chlamydia and Ureaplasma in pregnant patients. **Cefazolin** and other first generation cephalosporins are used after cesarean section for prophylaxis against bacterial infections (i.e. endomyometritis). **Gentamicin** is used in urinary tract infections caused by gram negative bacteria such as *Klebsiella-Enterobacter, Proteus, Pseudomonas*, and *Serratia*. **Penicillin** is used in the treatment of infections caused by group A & B streptococci, and *Treponema pallidum* (syphilis). **Penicillin** is no longer the drug of choice for gonorrhea since gonococci now show widespread resistance to penicillin. **Spectinomycin** can be used to treat gonorrhea in patients who are allergic to penicillins and cephalosporins. **Spiramycin** is the drug of choice for toxoplasmosis during pregnancy; the drug is not effective for other forms of the infection.

Dale, Infectious Disease, Chapter 22, pp 13-14.
DeCherney, 8th ed., pp 703-05, 762, 789-796.
Tierney, 38th ed., pp 707, 1383, 1467.

97

(Block 2: Item 47)

(H)

Psoriasis is a common skin disorder characterized by red, sharply defined plaques covered with silvery scales. These lesions are most often found on the elbows, knees, and scalp. Other sites of involvement include the palms, soles, glans penis and vulva. Psoriasis often affects the nails, causing fine pitting and onycholysis (separation of the nail plate from the nail bed). Although generally not used clinically, the "Auspitz sign" refers to the bleeding spots that appear when the scale is scraped off. Psoriasis has several variants including the plaque type (most common), eruptive or guttate psoriasis that often follows streptococcal pharyngitis, and pustular psoriasis. Psoriasis is hereditary and has several trigger factors. Minor trauma such as rubbing and scratching is a major factor (Koebner's phenomenon). Other triggers include infections, stress, and drugs. Climate also affects the expression of psoriasis: hot weather, sunlight, and humidity decrease the symptoms, while cold weather worsens the outcome. Psoriatic arthritis is one of the seronegative (negative rheumatoid factor) spondyloarthropathies, along with ankylosing spondylitis and Reiter's syndrome. Treatment options for psoriasis include minimizing scratching, topical steroids, topical tar preparations, topical or systemic retinoids, topical Vitamin D analogues, and UV light exposure.

Contact dermatitis is characterized by erythema, edema, and pruritus, often followed by vesicles and bullae, in an area exposed to an allergen. Weeping, crusting, and secondary infections are common. Four out of five cases are due to excessive exposure to irritants such as soaps, detergents, or organic solvents; this is known as irritant contact dermatitis. Other cases are due to contact with allergens such as poison ivy or poison oak; these are termed allergic contact dermatitis. **Atopic dermatitis** is a pruritic, exudative, or lichenified eruption commonly occurring on the face, neck, upper trunk, wrists, hands and in the antecubital and popliteal folds. Patients typically have a personal or family history of allergic manifestations (e.g., asthma). Atopic dermatitis tends to recur from adolescence to age 20. Pruritic 1-2 mm "tapioca" vesicles on the palms, soles and sides of fingers characterize **dyshidrotic eczema (dyshidrosis, pompholyx)**. The vesicles may merge and produce multiloculated blisters. It usually appears in the third decade and frequently recurs. **Lichen simplex chronicus** (circumscribed or localized neurodermatitis) presents as chronic itching of hyper-pigmented lichenified (exaggerated skin lines overlying a thickened, well-circumscribed scaly plaque) skin lesions. These lesions frequently occur in the nape of the neck, wrists, external surfaces of forearms, lower legs, popliteal and antecubital areas. **Nummular eczema** presents as numerous symmetrically distributed round plaques of dermatitis, most frequently involving the extremities. These lesions may be dry and scaly or oozing, and crusted. **Scabies** is characterized by pruritic vesicles and pustules in clusters, most commonly involving finger webs, palms and wrist creases. Mites, ova, and brown dots of feces from *Sarcoptes scabiei* infestation are noted on microscopic exam. Red papules or nodules are often seen on the penile glans and shaft. **Tinea corporis** often presents as ring-shaped lesions with advancing scaly borders and central clearing or scaly patches with distinct borders. It is typically on exposed skin surfaces or the trunk. Fungal hyphae would be demonstrated on microscopic examination of KOH-prepared scrapings.

Dale, Deramtology, Chapter 3, pp 1-12.
Farber, p 1.
Hay, 14th ed., p 354.
Tierney, 38th ed., pp 125-28, 132, 141, 143-45, 165.

98

(Block 2: Item 48)

(G)

Pityriasis rosea is a common, idiopathic disorder typically affecting those between the ages of 10 and 35. It is twice as common in women. Itching is common, but is generally mild. A larger lesion known as a "herald patch" usually precedes the appearance of a bilaterally symmetric eruption on the trunk and upper extremities by 1-2 weeks. The lesions are slightly raised, salmon colored, often with a fine wrinkled "cigarette paper" scale. The lesions tend to fall in cleavage planes producing a "Christmas tree" distribution. Not to worry, this is a self-limiting disorder that usually resolves after six to eight weeks. Pityriasis rosea can be easily confused with the roseola of secondary syphilis, which can be ruled out with appropriate serologic testing.

Dale, Dermatology, Chapter 2, p 1.

99

(Block 2: Item 49)

(I)

Lack of adequate sunlight (30 minutes total body, or 2 hours head exposure per week for infants), coupled with a low dietary intake may result in vitamin D deficiency. An infant who is exclusively breast-fed can acquire sufficient **vitamin D** from human milk only if the mother's vitamin D status is optimal (vitamin D deficiency in U.S. women is rare). The American Academy of Pediatrics (Policy statement, December 1997) recommends that vitamin D and iron only be given to select groups of infants younger than 6 months of age (vitamin D for infants whose mothers are vitamin-D deficient or those infants not exposed to adequate sunlight; iron for those who have low iron stores or anemia). Otherwise supplementation is required to avoid development of rickets.

Breast-feeding can provide optimal nutrition for an infant during the early months of life. Immunoactive factors in breast milk such as secretory IgA, lysozyme, lactoferrin, and macrophages protect against gastrointestinal and upper respiratory infections. Allergic diseases are less common in infants who are exclusively breast-fed. Also the relationship developed through breast-feeding is an important early maternal-infant interaction and provides for a source of security and comfort. Contraindications to breast-feeding include maternal tuberculosis, galactosemia in the infant, and maternal HIV infection. Compared to cow's milk and formulas, human milk contains less protein, more essential fatty acids, long chain unsaturated fatty acids such as docosahexaenoic acid, lower sodium and solute load, and a lower concentration of calcium, iron and zinc. However, due to better absorption of human milk, the infant receives adequate quantities of these nutrients despite lower absolute intakes. After the age of 6 months it is recommended that a source of iron such as fortified cereal, meat or supplement be added to the diet.

A breast-fed infant should be supplemented with: **vitamin B_1** if the mother is alcoholic or malnourished (although some pediatricians counsel against alcoholic mothers breastfeeding), and **vitamin B_{12}** if the mother is vegan. **Vitamin K** is usually given at birth. **Calcium deficiency** can occur in premature infants and lactating adolescents in addition to patients with steatorrhea. This may result in decreased bone density and rickets. **Folic acid** deficiency is seen in prematurity, breast-fed infants of folate-deficient mothers, infants fed unsupplemented cow's milk or goat's milk, patients with kwashiorkor, sprue, celiac diseases, and infants on medication such as phenytoin. It may also be deficient in children with increased requirements secondary to chronic hemolytic anemias, diarrhea, malignancy, and infection. **Pyridoxine (vitamin B_6)** deficiency is seen in premature infants, in those treated with drugs such as isoniazid, and in those fed by heat-treated formulas. **Vitamin C** deficiency is seen in prematurity, in infants whose mothers received excessive amounts of vitamin C during pregnancy or avoided fresh fruits and vegetables, and in those infants fed formula and pasteurized cow milk. **Vitamin A** deficiency occurs in prematurity, intravenous nutritional states, protein-energy malnutrition, and fat malabsorption syndromes such as giardiasis and cystic fibrosis. **Vitamin E** deficiency occurs in prematurity, cholestatic liver disease, pancreatic insufficiency of cystic fibrosis, abetalipoproteinemia, and short bowel syndrome.

Hay, 14th ed., pp 256-62.
http://www.aap.org/policy/re9729.html

100

(Block 2: Item 50)

(D, I, J)

Cystic fibrosis is characterized by defective chloride conduction across the apical membrane of epithelial cells secondary to a mutation in the cystic fibrosis trans-membrane conductance regulator (CFTR). 90% of patients with cystic fibrosis eventually display some evidence of pancreatic insufficiency caused by partial or complete occlusion of ductal and saccular structures by inspissated secretions. Pancreatic insufficiency, can in turn, cause malnutrition and deficiencies of **lipid-soluble vitamins, such as D, A, K, and E**.

Dale, Gastroenterology, Chapter 5, pp 13-14.

101

(Block 3: Item 1)

(D)

Systemic scleroderma is characterized by skin changes and multisystem involvement. Organs commonly affected include lungs, gastrointestinal tract, heart and kidneys. Organ damage is either caused by ischemia from vascular lesions or an increase in local collagen accumulation. It is usually seen in women between the ages of 20 and 50. Renal involvement, seen in 20-50% of patients with diffuse scleroderma, involves obliterative arterial lesions of the interlobular arteries, in addition to concentric "onion skin" thickening of the vessel walls resulting from proliferation of smooth muscle cells in the media.

"Scleroderma renal crisis" is characterized by the sudden onset of renal failure (progressive within days to weeks). These patients typically have mild proteinuria with few cells or casts (secondary to the noninflammatory nature of scleroderma). Hematuria secondary to ischemia-induced glomerular necrosis may also be noted. The activation of the renin-angiotensin system can produce marked elevations in blood pressure and is a factor in the pathogenesis of renal scleroderma. If **antihypertensive therapy with ACE inhibitors** is started before irreversible vascular injury has occurred, renal failure may be prevented. However, patients, who progress to renal failure with—(1) uremic symptoms such as pericarditis, encephalopathy or coagulopathy, (2) fluid overload unresponsive to diuresis, (3) refractory hyperkalemia, (4) severe metabolic acidosis (pH < 7.20), or (5) neurologic symptoms such as seizures or neuropathy—require dialysis. Our patient has markedly elevated potassium (6.2 mEq/L); with concomitant renal insufficiency, hemodialysis is the appropriate treatment option. **Hemodialysis** is the preferred method of dialysis in an acutely hospitalized patient with vascular access. 50% of scleroderma patients, who are on short-term dialysis, eventually manage to get off dialysis.

Intravenous administration of morphine would not address the underlying renal failure. Also since the patient's renal failure is not secondary to prerenal causes, **fluid administration** would not help. Finally **peritoneal dialysis** in a patient with scleroderma may become useful if the patient progresses to require chronic dialysis, if lack of vascular access makes hemodialysis technically difficult, or if the patient requires more autonomy (hemodialysis requires 3-4 hours per session, three times a week).

Dale, Nephrology, Chapter 7, pp 6-7.
Tierney, 38th ed., pp 846, 879.

102

(Block 3: Item 2)

(C)

Compression of the **median nerve** as it passes through the carpal tunnel, formed by carpal bones inferiorly and the carpal ligament superiorly, causes the carpal tunnel syndrome. The motor components of median nerve affected past the point of obstruction in the carpal tunnel include thenar muscles (abductor pollicis brevis, opponens pollicis, flexor pollicis brevis) and lumbricals 1 and 2. The sensory area affected is the posterior and anterior surface of the first three and a half digits and the corresponding palmar area. Carpal tunnel syndrome is characterized by episodic numbness in the median nerve sensory distribution, frequently occurring at night and during flexion or extension of the wrist. Vigorous shaking of the hand often alleviates the symptoms. Thenar muscle weakness may be noted, especially in the elderly. "Tinel's sign" is transient paresthesia in the median innervated digits after percussion of the median nerve at the wrist. "Phalen's sign" describes exacerbation of symptoms secondary to forced extension or flexion of the wrist for one to two minutes, which is relieved by hanging the arm loosely at the side without wrist angulation. Carpal tunnel syndrome may be treated by splinting, glucocorticoid injections or surgical sectioning of the carpal ligament.

The **axillary, brachial cutaneous, radial and ulnar nerves** do not traverse the carpal tunnel or innervate the thenar group of muscles.

Dale, Neurology, Chapter 2, pp 5-6.
Pansky, 6th ed., p 323.

103

(Block 3: Item 3)

(C)

Late antepartum hemorrhage is defined as vaginal bleeding that occurs after 20 weeks of gestation. The differential diagnosis includes placenta previa, placental abruption, uterine rupture, and vasa previa. Placenta previa refers to implantation of the placenta in the lower uterine segment in the zone of effacement and dilation of the cervix. This causes an obstruction to the descent of the presenting part. Placenta previa occurs in 1 out of 200 deliveries, is usually diagnosed in the second trimester, and may be marginal, partial or total depending on the degree of obstruction. Only 20% of all cases of placenta previa cause total obstruction. Patients typically present with bright red vaginal bleeding and relatively little or no pain. Increasing maternal age, multiparity and prior uterine scars are prior risk factors. Placental abruption, separation of the placenta from the site of uterine implantation before delivery of the fetus, occurs in up to 10% of all deliveries. It may be mild (slight vaginal bleeding, no fetal heart rate abnormalities and no evidence of shock or coagulopathy), moderate (moderate vaginal bleeding, shock and fetal distress), or severe (extensive vaginal bleeding, tetanic uterus, maternal shock, fetal demise and maternal coagulopathy). The patient typically presents with pain and increased uterine tone. Prior history of abruption, maternal hypertension, cigarette or cocaine use, increasing maternal age and multiparity are risk factors. **Ultrasonography** is used in the diagnosis of placenta previa and placental abruption, it also allows for assessment of fetal well being, estimation of gestational age, and localization of amniotic fluid. It should be performed in the labor and delivery area with interval monitoring of the fetal heart rate. **Amniocentesis to evaluate pulmonary maturity** would only be indicated if premature delivery was expected. Should this become necessary, it would be done during ultrasonography.

Rupture of the uterus presents with increased suprapubic pain and tenderness, sudden cessation of uterine contractions during labor with a "tearing" sensation, vaginal bleeding, and disappearance of fetal heart tones. It occurs in approximately 1in 1500 deliveries usually in patients with previous cesarean scars or history of trauma. Vasa previa refers to placement of the fetal vessels associated with velamentous insertion of the cord in the lower uterine segment within the path of the presenting part. In this condition the vessels may be disrupted during labor or rupture of membranes resulting in rapid bleeding and fetal exsanguination. It should be considered if the fetus is tachycardic soon after rupture of membranes. In the **"double set-up examination"** the patient is completely set up for cesarean section, with the exception of anesthetic administration. A thorough vaginal exam with a speculum is then conducted. It was previously believed that if the placenta was not visualized during this procedure, placenta previa could be ruled out. This examination is now believed to be a very inaccurate and dangerous method of diagnosis compared to ultrasonography and cesarean delivery without vaginal examination.

Evaluation of **umbilical blood flow using Doppler waveform analyses** may be helpful in identifying a fetus at risk for intrauterine growth retardation. This imaging modality has no role in antepartum hemorrhage. The decision to proceed with **immediate cesarean delivery,** continued labor, or expectant management depends on the status of the mother, fetus and placenta. Cesarean delivery is the method of choice in every type of placenta previa. In placental abruption it is performed when the distressed fetus has a reasonable chance of survival but delivery is not imminent. Cesarean delivery is also preferred in uncontrollable maternal hemorrhage.

DeCherney, 8th ed., pp 285, 399-408, 506.

104

(Block 3: Item 4)

(B)

Sulfamethoxazole therapy is associated with generalized skin eruptions, skin rash, urticaria, **photosensitivity** and pruritus. Drug eruptions may present as urticarial, morbilliform (resembling the eruption of measles), scarlatiniform (resembling the rash of scarlet fever), or bullous lesions. Urticaria may present within minutes after drug administration but most reactions appear after 1 to 2 weeks. Eruptions may occur in patients who have received the drug for long periods, and may continue for days after the drug has been stopped. While many drugs including sulfamethoxazole may cause eruptions, photosensitivity is typically caused by Psoralens, tetracyclines, thiazides and sulfonamides.

Reaction to a jellyfish sting would be expected immediately after contact and only on exposed surfaces. Patches of erythema, exudation, and scaling, sometimes forming larger plaques characterize **eczema** usually seen in infants and children. ***Salmonella typhi***, the cause of typhoid fever, presents with malaise, headache, crampy abdominal pain, distention and constipation, followed in 48 hours by diarrhea, high fever and encephalopathy. The associated rash known as "rose spots" is present in 10-15% of affected children and appears in crops during the second week of disease. These are erythematous maculopapular 2-3 mm lesions that fade on pressure and are typically found on the chest and trunk. *S. typhi* is transmitted through ingestion of contaminated food (poultry, eggs, and dairy products) or water. **Enterotoxigenic *E. coli*** causes a secretory watery diarrhea by adhering to enterocytes and secreting one or more plasmid encoded enterotoxins. One of these toxins resembles cholera toxin in structure, function and mechanism of action. By binding to a regulatory subunit of adenyl cyclase in enterocytes, the toxin causes increased cAMP production and an outpouring of NaCl and water into the lumen of the small bowel. The symptoms are usually mild and self-limited without significant fever or systemic toxicity; a skin rash is not noted.

Hay, 14th ed., pp 358, 1030, 1034.

105

(Block 3: Item 5)

(A)

Marfan's syndrome is a connective tissue disorder that has widespread physical abnormalities. Patients with this syndrome present with disproportionate growth (lengthened wingspan and arachnodactyly), joint hyperextensibility, lens dislocation, and dilation of the aortic root. The defect in fibrillin, a structural component of elastin associated microfibrils, leads to disruption of collagen and elastin fibers in vessels and valves, thereby causing dilation, dissection and rupture of the aorta and prolapse of the valves. Cardiovascular abnormalities cause many fatalities in these patients. Patients should be followed by annual echocardiograms and if the diameter of the aortic root exceeds 6 cm causing significant **aortic regurgitation**, aortic valve replacement is indicated. Mitral valve prolapse accompanied by severe mitral regurgitation may also be noted in patients with Marfan's syndrome. Aortic regurgitation presents with wide pulse pressure, an enlarged left ventricle, and a diastolic murmur best heard along the left sternal border. ECG typically shows left ventricular hypertrophy, and chest X-ray shows left ventricular dilation.

Atrial septal defects (ASD) are typically asymptomatic until middle age. Important physical exam findings are right ventricular lift, widely split and fixed S_2, and a grade I-III/VI systolic ejection murmur at the pulmonary area. ECG reveals right ventricular conduction delay while chest X-ray usually shows dilated pulmonary arteries and increased vascularity. ASD is not a feature of Marfan's syndrome. **Coarctation of the aorta** may cause severe heart failure in infants, but children and adults are usually asymptomatic, presenting only with hypertension. Patients typically have absent or weak femoral pulses and higher systolic pressures in the upper extremities compared to the lower extremities. The characteristic murmur is systolic and heard in the back. ECG typically shows left ventricular hypertrophy while chest X-ray shows "rib notching" (secondary to increased collateral flow). **Ebstein's anomaly** is a congenital defect of the tricuspid valve consisting of downward leaflet malinsertion. Patients span a spectrum from asymptomatic to those with congestive heart failure secondary to significant valvular regurgitation and low right ventricular output. Tricuspid regurgitation associated with Ebstein's anomaly typically produces a loud S_1 and a harsh systolic murmur along the lower left sternal border increasing in intensity during and after inspiration. Patients with **mitral stenosis** present with dyspnea, orthopnea, and paroxysmal nocturnal dyspnea. Pregnancy or the onset of atrial fibrillation often precipitates their symptoms. The physical exam demonstrates a prominent first heart sound, opening snap and apical crescendo rumble. ECG typically shows left atrial enlargement.

Daldah, pp 427-32.
Dale, Cardiovascular Medicine, Chapter 12, p 4.
Tierney, 38th ed., pp 346-47, 349-50, 356.

106

(Block 3: Item 6)

(D)

Bias is defined as a systematic error in a study that leads to distortion of results. It can occur in any type of study but is of particular concern in observational studies, because the lack of complete randomization in such studies increases the chance that study groups differ in important characteristics. There are three main categories of bias: selection bias, information bias, and confounding. In **selection bias**, the selection process itself may alter the chance that a relationship between the exposure and disease of interest will be detected. Volunteers for a study may differ from those who do not volunteer in age, race, economic status, education level and gender. Volunteers may also be healthier than those who do not participate.

Information bias describes random or systematic inaccuracy in measurement. Two common types of information bias are recall bias and **interviewer (observer) bias**. In recall bias, subjects may have difficulty remembering previous activities and exposures. In interviewer bias, results may be influenced by how the information is collected. If they are aware of the hypothesis, interviewers may intentionally or unintentionally influence the responses of the subjects. Confounding refers to the effect of a third variable or correlate on the interaction between the exposure and disease of interest. The variable is typically associated with the disease of interest in the absence of exposure, and is also associated with the exposure but not as a result of being exposed. **Placebo effect** was best described by Haygarth in 1801: "The wonderful and powerful influence of the passions of the mind upon the state and disorders of the body" are "too often overlooked in the cure of diseases." To reduce introduction of bias due to patients' and clinicians' perceptions, study subjects and interviewers are **blinded**. The "blinded" person does not know the treatment assignment. **Randomization** determines treatment group assignment based on probability alone and removes bias introduced by physician or patient preferences. It also maximizes the probability that the two groups will be similar in background characteristics that may influence the study outcome. All of the possible answers to this question could account for the observation reported. Given the study design, however, self-selection bias is by far the most likely.

Greenberg, 2nd ed., pp 91, 93, 136-41.

107

(Block 3: Item 7)

(E)

Ventricular septal defect, the most common congenital cardiac anomaly in infants, may involve the membranous or muscular portions of the ventricular septum. A large VSD causes a left to right shunt that results in volume overload and ventricular hypertrophy. Infants typically present with congestive heart failure 2-3 months after birth. The characteristic murmur is pansystolic. Ventricular septal defects may be complicated by "Eisenmenger's Syndrome" secondary to chronic volume overload and ventricular hypertrophy; this increases right-sided pressures and causes pulmonary hypertension, eventually leading to reversal of blood flow through the shunt (and resultant cyanosis).

Acute bronchiolitis typically presents with fever, tachypnea, cough, rhinorrhea, and expiratory wheezing. Nasal flaring, respiratory distress, cyanosis, retractions and rales may also be present. Respiratory syncytial virus is the most common etiologic agent. Not only do the acute effects of bronchiolitis cause concern, but also the development of chronic airway hyperreactivity or asthma are chronic complications. **Allergy to formula** must present with a temporal relationship between ingestion of a suspected food and onset of allergic symptoms with most reactions occurring in minutes to 2 hours after ingestion. Symptoms can be either immediate or delayed and may involve: (1) GI tract (nausea, vomiting, diarrhea, abdominal cramps), (2) respiratory (wheezing, coughing, rhinorrhea, tongue/pharynx, and upper airway pruritus/angioedema), and most commonly, (3) skin (urticaria, angioedema, flushing). **Atrial septal defects** are typically asymptomatic until middle age. Sometimes infants with ASDs may have slow weight gain and frequent lower respiratory infections. Important physical exam findings are right ventricular lift, widely split and fixed S_2, and a grade I-III/VI systolic ejection murmur at the pulmonary area. ECG reveals right ventricular conduction delay while chest X-ray usually shows dilated pulmonary arteries and increased vascularity. **Pulmonary hypertension** in the infant may be caused by increased pulmonary blood flow with only a slight increase in pulmonary vascular resistance. This may occur secondary to a shunt such as patent ductus arteriosus. In such a case the patient would present with the shunt findings (bounding pulses, widened pulse pressure, narrow and split second heart sound, and a rough machinery murmur at the left sternal border of the second intercostal space that radiates to the back) in addition to an accentuated pulmonary component of S_2 and cyanosis.

Dale, Cardiovascular Medicine, Chapter 15, p 5.
Hay, 14th ed., pp 57, 346-47, 431-32, 485, 940.

108

(Block 3: Item 8)

(B)

A deficiency of **folate** in a pregnant woman may lead to an increased risk of neural tube defects including anencephaly and spina bifida in the infant. This risk may be reduced by folic acid supplementation given before and after the time of conception. Folate is found in green leafy vegetables and citrus fruits. Patients most susceptible to folate deficiency are those receiving anticonvulsants or oral contraceptives (secondary to impaired absorption or metabolism) in addition to pregnant patients who have increased requirements due to increased hematopoiesis.

Calcium intake should be increased to 1.5 g/d towards the end of pregnancy and during lactation. If maternal intake is inadequate, skeletal demineralization occurs until the nutritional requirements of the fetus or nursing baby are met. Vitamin and mineral preparations are commonly used during pregnancy but their use should not be substituted for adequate food intake. **Vitamin A** is essential for retinal function, cell growth and differentiation, and normal wound healing and is found in pigmented vegetables. **Vitamin D** is found in milk or other processed foods and its deficiency is rarely seen in the United States. Adequate intake of vitamin D is necessary for normal calcium uptake and bone formation. **Vitamin B_{12}** belongs to the cobalamin family and is essential for normal hematopoiesis. In pregnancy, vitamin B_{12} supplements are beneficial for vegetarian patients and those with known megaloblastic anemia.

Dale, Neurology, Chapter 3, p 12.
DeCherney, 8th ed., p 197.

109

(Block 3: Item 9)

(E)

It is difficult to distinguish hematologic abnormalities caused by alcohol itself from those caused by associated diseases such as liver disease, folate or iron deficiency, variceal bleeding or hypersplenism (with trapping of leukocytes and platelets). Daily consumption of approximately 80 grams of alcohol may produce macrocytosis, vacuolization of proerythroblasts and thrombocytopenia in addition to profound suppression of hematopoiesis. In addition to **marrow suppression**, this patient manifests some symptoms of alcoholic hepatitis. Typical symptoms are anorexia, nausea, hepatomegaly, jaundice, abdominal pain and tenderness, splenomegaly, ascites, fever, and encephalopathy. As seen in this patient, AST is usually elevated but rarely above 300 U. AST is often greater than ALT by a factor of 2. The longer the duration of drinking the higher the chance of developing alcoholic hepatitis and cirrhosis. The patient is also going through alcohol withdrawal that typically presents with anxiety, decreased cognition, tremulousness and elevated vital signs. This may progress to delirium tremens—an acute organic psychosis that manifests 25-72 hours after the last drink. It is characterized by mental confusion, tremor, sensory hyperacuity, visual hallucinations, autonomic hyperactivity, diaphoresis, dehydration, hypokalemia, hypomagnesemia, seizures and cardiovascular abnormalities.

Drug metabolism by the liver is altered by alcohol consumption, especially in the setting of alcoholic hepatitis. Thus the patient is at increased risk for developing **adverse drug reactions** secondary to interaction with alcohol. Drugs commonly causing pancytopenia include chloramphenicol, phenylbutazone, gold salts, sulfonamides, phenytoin, carbamazepine, quinacrine, and tolbutamide. **Hypersplenism** refers to trapping of erythrocytes, leukocytes and platelets in an enlarged spleen. In this question however, there is no mention of splenomegaly on physical exam (albeit a poor test for detecting an enlarged spleen). **Myelophthisic marrow** refers to the replacement of marrow elements by an infiltrative process, such as malignancy or infection. Such a process would be unlikely in a patient with an acute course. **Peripheral destruction of cells** is characteristic of hemolytic anemias such as thrombotic thrombocytopenic purpura (TTP), hemolytic uremic syndrome (HUS) and disseminated intravascular coagulation (DIC). TTP typically presents with microangiopathic hemolytic anemia, thrombocytopenia, neurologic and renal abnormalities, fever, elevated serum LDH and normal coagulation tests. HUS presents with microangiopathic hemolytic anemia, thrombocytopenia, renal failure, elevated serum LDH, normal coagulation tests, and no neurologic abnormalities (in contrast to TTP). DIC usually manifests secondary to an underlying serious illness. It presents with microangiopathic hemolytic anemia, low fibrinogen, thrombocytopenia, high fibrin degradation products, and prolonged prothrombin time.

Dale, Hematology, Chapter 3, p 1.
Tierney, 38th ed., pp 501-02, 522-32, 649, 1034.

110

(Block 3: Item 10)

(B)

Patients with **chronic lymphocytic leukemia** (CLL), a malignant clonal disorder of predominantly B cells (5% T cell origin), often present with leukocytosis, discovered incidentally on routine CBC. They also have hypogammaglobulinemia and abnormal immunity. CLL is most often seen in the elderly and is usually indolent with progressive accumulation of long-lived lymphocytes, which are immunocompetent but respond poorly to antigenic stimulation. CLL manifests clinically as immunosuppression, bone marrow failure and organ infiltration by lymphocytes. It is also associated with autoimmune hemolytic anemia (5-10% of cases) and idiopathic thrombocytopenic purpura (ITP). Physical examination may reveal nontender adenopathy and moderate splenomegaly. Pancytopenia, impressive nodal enlargement, organomegaly and recurrent infections may be part of the presentation. The patient's anemia and thrombocytopenia in this case are most likely caused by autoimmune hemolysis rather than marrow infiltration alone since the peripheral smear shows several spherocytes and reticulocytes. However, a positive Coombs test would be required for definitive proof.

Myelofibrosis (agnogenic myeloid metaplasia) is a myeloproliferative disorder presenting with splenomegaly, teardrop poikilocytosis, giant abnormal platelets and hypercellular bone marrow with reticulin or collagen fibrosis. Patients typically present with fatigue secondary to anemia or abdominal fullness due to splenomegaly. **Chronic myelogenous leukemia** usually features a strikingly elevated white blood cell count, markedly left-shifted myeloid series but progressively fewer promyelocytes and blasts, and the presence of Philadelphia chromosome or bcr-abl gene. Patients typically present in middle age with complaints of fatigue, night sweats, low grade fever and abdominal fullness due to splenomegaly. Patients with infectious mononucleosis secondary to **Epstein-Barr virus infection** may have fever, adenopathy, sore throat, maculopapular rash resembling rubella, splenomegaly and tonsillar exudates. Laboratory tests reveal atypical lymphocytes in blood smears, heterophil agglutination and a positive Monospot test. **Hodgkin's disease** has a bimodal age distribution with a peak in the 20s and a second peak over age 50. Most patients present with painless lymphadenopathy, fever, weight loss, drenching night sweats and generalized pruritus. Patients often complain of pain in the involved lymph nodes following alcohol ingestion. **Left-shifted granulocytosis** is leukocytosis with a predominance of neutrophils and band forms. This is a typical laboratory feature of bacterial infections and, at times, can closely imitate the left shifted myeloid production of chronic myelogenous leukemia mentioned above.

Dale, Hematology, Chapter 8, pp 16-17.
Tierney, 38th ed., pp 507-09, 517, 1260.

111

(Block 3: Item 11)

(F)

This patient presents with weight loss, shortness of breath, cough, a 44 pack-year history of smoking, a supraclavicular node, and evidence of a mass lesion in the lung and the adrenal on imaging. A neoplastic process is the most likely cause of these symptoms and findings. Lung cancer is the leading cause of death in men and since 1985 in women in the United States (almost 1/3 of all cancer deaths.) Lung cancer is associated with a low cure rate since most patients are identified when the disease is already advanced. There is a strong association between cigarette smoking and lung cancer. Lung cancers have been classified in two major categories: small cell lung cancer (SCLC) and **non-small cell lung cancer (NSCLC)**. Small cell undifferentiated lung cancer is comprised of malignant cells of neuroectodermal origin and is often associated with paraneoplastic syndromes. Characteristically, it has early hematogenous dissemination and is rarely cured by surgery. It is very sensitive to chemotherapy and radiation. Cure is possible with the early combined use of combination chemotherapy and radiation. All other epithelial lung malignancies are termed non-small cell lung cancer (NSCLC), with the major types being: (1) squamous cell carcinoma, (2) adenocarcinoma, and (3) large cell undifferentiated carcinoma. Characteristically, NSCLC are treated more effectively with surgery (when diagnosed early enough, Stage I and II) and are poorly responsive to radiation and chemotherapy. Smoking is the major cause of all epithelial lung cancers (small cell and non-small cell). **Adenocarcinoma** is the only histology increasing in frequency among non-smokers. In the past, <10% of patients with adenocarcinoma were nonsmokers; currently, approximately 25% of adenocarcinoma patients are nonsmokers. The reasons for this increase are unclear. The extensive history of smoking and the presence of adrenal metastasis in this patient point to NSCLC as the most likely diagnosis.

Patients with **lymphomas** typically present with painless lymphadenopathy. If symptoms are present, they include fever, drenching night sweats, and weight loss. Isolated sites of extranodal disease (skin, gastrointestinal tract) may be found, but a parenchymal lung mass would be rare compared to the incidence of primary bronchogenic carcinoma in smokers. Tissue biopsy is diagnostic. **Lung abscesses** usually occur in patients with predisposition to aspiration or poor dental hygiene. These patients present with fever, weight loss, malaise, and foul-smelling sputum. **Lung mesotheliomas** are tumors arising from the surface lining of the pleura. They may be diffuse (75% of cases, malignant) or localized (25% of cases, usually benign). Mesotheliomas are three times more common in men and are associated with exposure to asbestos. Mean age at onset of symptoms is 60 years. Symptoms include shortness of breath, non-pleuritic chest pain, and weight loss. X-ray reveals nodular, irregular unilateral pleural thickening, pleural effusion, and evidence for asbestos exposure manifest as calcified pleural plaques. Women at risk for development of **breast cancer** are those with delayed childbearing, family history of breast cancer, and mammary dysplasia on prior biopsy. Early findings include a single, nontender, firm mass with ill-defined margins or mammographic microcalcifications. Late findings are skin or nipple retraction, axillary lymphadenopathy, breast enlargement, redness, edema, pain and fixation of the mass to skin or chest wall. The most common sites of breast cancer metastasis are lungs, bone, liver, and soft tissue (i.e. regional nodes and skin). Brain, adrenal, ovary, and other non-hepatic intraabdominal sites are less common and seen primarily in far-advanced disease. **Multiple endocrine neoplasias** (MEN) are several syndromes with multiple gland involvement. MEN 1 is the most common and presents with hyperparathyroidism, pancreatic islet cell tumors and pituitary adenomas. Medullary thyroid carcinoma, pheochromocytomas and hyperparathyroidism characterize MEN 2a. MEN 2b is the triad of medullary thyroid carcinomas, pheochromocytomas and mucosal neuromas. **Sarcoidosis** usually occurs in the 30-40s predominantly in African American women and Northern European Caucasians. Patients present with malaise, fever and dyspnea. Bilateral hilar and paratracheal lymphadenopathy is the characteristic finding on chest X-ray. Laboratory findings include leukopenia, eosinophilia, elevated erythrocyte sedimentation rate, hypercalcemia, hypercalciuria, and elevated angiotensin converting enzyme levels. **Tuberculosis** typically presents with fatigue, weight loss, fever, night sweats, cough, and pulmonary infiltrates on chest X-ray. Laboratory findings include positive tuberculin skin reaction, acid-fast bacilli (AFB) on smear of sputum, or sputum culture positive for *Mycobacterium tuberculosis.*

Dale, Oncology, Chapter 6, pp 1-8.
Tierney, 38th ed., pp 288-91, 304-05, 308-09, 515-16, 681-86, 1114-16.

112

(Block 3: Item 12)

(D)

Normal grieving following the death of a loved one or any other serious loss may include somatic symptoms such as sighing respirations, exhaustion, gastrointestinal symptoms of all kinds, restlessness, yawning and choking. Feelings of guilt are common especially early in the grieving process. An intense focus on the image of the lost person, manifesting as having mental conversations with them, sensing their presence and auditory, visual or tactile hallucinations involving them may be present. The affected person may also be irritable and hostile. This process typically lasts 1-3 months but may vary depending on the individual situation. Resolution is signaled by reappearance of normal functioning, the capacity to experience pleasure and the ability to enter new relationships.

Conversion disorder is characterized by conversion of psychic conflict into physical symptoms in body parts innervated by the sensorimotor system. The typical somatic manifestation is paralysis. **Generalized anxiety disorder** is the most common anxiety disorder, usually occurring at age 20-35 years with a slight predominance in women. The patient presents with disabling apprehension, anxiety, worry, irritability, hypervigilance, insomnia, and somatic complaints for at least one month. **Major depressive disorder** is characterized by periods of serious mood depression with loss of interest and pleasure, withdrawal from daily activities, feelings of guilt, inability to concentrate, cognitive dysfunction, anxiety, chronic fatigue, worthlessness, somatic complaints and loss of sexual drive. Sadness and grief are normal responses to loss, but depression is not. Normal grief is usually accompanied by intact self-esteem whereas **pathologic grief** is characterized by a severe sense of guilt and worthlessness, or by the presence of significant suicidal ideation of psychotic symptoms.

Dale, Psychiatry, Chapter 1, pp 2-3.
Tierney, 38th ed., pp 995, 999, 1016-17.

113

(Block 3: Item 13)

(A)

Acute stress disorder, a new diagnosis in the DSM IV, describes a syndrome of severe dissociation (amnesia, derealization, detachment, reduced awareness), intrusion (recurrent images, thoughts, dreams, illusions), avoidance (especially of stimuli arousing recollection of stressor), and hyperarousal symptoms (anxiety, difficulty sleeping) immediately following a traumatic event. Only a minority of trauma victims suffers this degree of symptoms. These patients are at risk of poor coping and can progress to post traumatic stress disorder if symptoms last over one month.

Agoraphobia or fear of being in situations from which escape might be difficult (open places and public areas), is often associated with severe panic attacks. Patients often develop agoraphobia in early adult life. **Generalized anxiety disorder** is the most common anxiety disorder, usually occurring at age 20-35 years with a slight predominance in women. The patient presents with disabling apprehension, anxiety, worry, irritability, hypervigilance, insomnia, and somatic complaints for at least one month. **Hypothyroidism** is not likely in the setting of a normal TSH (0.5-5 μU/mL); furthermore, the patient's symptoms of tachycardia and anxiety are more likely in hyperthyroidism than hypothyroidism. These symptoms may be part of her stress disorder, due to too much levothyroxine, or secondary to a beta-agonist asthma inhaler. **Panic disorder** is characterized by short lived, recurrent unexpected attacks of intense anxiety accompanied by marked physiological manifestations. Agoraphobia may also be present. Symptoms include dyspnea, tachycardia, palpitations, headaches, dizziness, paresthesias, choking, smothering feelings, nausea, bloating, and feelings of impending doom.

Gabbard, pp 1522-23.
Tierney, 38th ed., 995-96.

114

(Block 3: Item 14)

(C)

Acute otitis media (OM) is a very common condition of young children; bacteria ascend from the nasopharynx to the normally sterile middle ear and cause infection. Children have shorter eustachian tubes than adults, which allow bacteria and viruses an easier route to the middle ear. The pathogenesis may involve abnormal eustachian tube function or obstruction caused by viral or allergic nasopharyngitis. Classic presenting signs include pain and hearing loss. Patients may also present with fever, tympanic membrane perforation and otorrhea. On examination a bulging membrane with impaired mobility and obstruction of the bony landmarks are noted. OM is caused by viruses (30% of cases), *S. pneumoniae* (33%), non-typeable strains of ***H. influenzae*** (20%), and *M. catarrhalis* (6-10%). Other less common pathogens include *S. pyogenes,* ***S. aureus,*** *Chlamydia trachomatis*, gram-negative enteric organisms and anaerobic organisms. Pathogens responsible for OM generally respond to amoxicillin or trimethoprim-sulfamethoxazole. The dose of amoxicillin in OM is very important. Approximately 40% of *S. pneumoniae* OM are intermediate-highly resistant to amoxicillin. High dose amoxicillin (60-90 mg/kg/day) will be effective against these resistant organisms, whereas Augmentin or macrolides will not. Unfortunately, most strains of non-typeable *H. influenzae* and *M. catarrhalis* are beta-lactamase positive. No response after 72 hours of amoxicillin merits treatment with ampicillin-clavulanic acid, a second- or third-generation cephalosporin, or a macrolide antibiotic.

Dale, Infectious Disease, Chapter 19, pp 5-6.
Hay, 14th ed., pp 394-96.

115

(Block 3: Item 15)

(D)

A **"hot flash"** is a vasomotor response caused by decreasing estrogen levels. Estradiol levels gradually decline during the premenopausal stage of a woman's life; the decrease in the intermenstrual cycle is due to a shortened follicular phase. Typically, a hot flash presents as an awareness of heat, or pressure in the head, followed in 45-60 seconds by warmth and often sweating in the face, neck, and chest. Less commonly, patients complain also of weakness, fatigue, faintness and vertigo. These episodes are typically accompanied by a 2-4°C rise in surface temperature and 0.2-0.3°C fall in core temperature. Hot flashes are treated with estrogen replacement. The duration of symptoms varies from momentary to as long as ten minutes, with an average length of 4 minutes. The frequency varies from 1-2/hour to 1-2/week. None of the other choices offered produce the combination of short duration, and specific upper body distribution associated with hot flashes.

Paraneoplastic symptoms of a **carcinoid tumor** (carcinoid syndrome) include facial flushing, edema of the head and neck, abdominal cramps and diarrhea, bronchospasm, cardiac lesions (tricuspid stenosis, pulmonary stenosis, pulmonary regurgitation), telangiectasias, and increased urinary 5-HIAA. **Hyperthyroidism** frequently presents with sweating, tremor, anxiety, loose stools, heat intolerance, irritability, fatigue, weakness, menstrual irregularity, tachycardia, warm, moist skin, stare, and weight loss (although 10-15% of patients may actually experience weight gain probably from decreased activity secondary to fatigue). **Generalized anxiety disorder** is the most common anxiety disorder, usually occurring at age 20-35 years with a slight predominance in women. The patient presents with disabling apprehension, anxiety, worry, irritability, hypervigilance, insomnia, and somatic complaints for at least one month. **Excessive caffeine ingestion** would have periodic symptoms that follow ingestion of coffee (or other caffeinated drinks) closely. It would not have any specific body site distribution.

Dale, Endocrinology, Chapter 3, p 13.
DeCherney, 8th ed., p 1034.
Tierney, 38th ed., pp 97, 995, 1074.

116

(Block 3: Item 16)

(D)

Papilledema is bilateral optic disc swelling secondary to increased intracranial pressure. Headaches are frequently seen in patients with increased intracranial pressure. In patients also presenting with fevers, lethargy, nausea and vomiting, CNS infection is likely and must be ruled out. However, in the setting of increased intracranial pressure, **CT or MR imaging** is indicated prior to proceeding to lumbar puncture since a mass lesion must be excluded. Rapid decompression of the intracranial pressure by lumbar puncture in such patients may lead to herniation of the brain (through the foramen magnum) and death. The source of the CNS infection causing papilledema in this child is direct extension of sinus infection through the frontal bone into the intracranial space to produce meningitis and epidural, subdural, or parenchymal abscess. Causes of chronic sinusitis include mucosal inflammation secondary to allergic rhinitis leading to obstruction, anatomic variations such as septal deviation, or poor host resistance (Kartagener's syndrome, immune defects, and cystic fibrosis). Anaerobic or staphylococcal organisms are most often responsible.

Measurement of serum ammonia level would be helpful if one was considering hepatic encephalopathy as a possible etiology for the patient's lethargy and CNS symptoms. Since the possibility of cirrhosis and portal hypertension in this child is low, this test is not indicated. **X-ray films of the sinuses** would confirm the original diagnosis of chronic sinusitis, but would not offer any information regarding intracranial lesions. **Electroencephalography** is helpful in the assessment of patients who have had seizures at the time of presentation. In cases of infection the changes would be nonspecific and characterized by generalized slowing. In specific cases such as HSV infection, focal activity may be seen early in the course and may be one of the earliest diagnostic markers. EEG may also show focal slowing over regions of abscesses. However in this case the information it would provide would not be as specific and useful as that provided by a CT scan. After a mass lesion has been excluded by proper imaging, a **lumbar puncture** would be indicated to confirm infection by culture and to direct specific antibiotic therapy by providing sensitivity data.

Fauci, 14th ed., pp 167, 2281.
Hay, 14th ed., pp 407-08, 674.

117

(Block 3: Item 17)

(A)

The liver is the most common site of *Entamoeba histolytica* infection outside of the intestine. **Amebic liver abscess** caused by *E. histolytica* typically presents with fever and right upper quadrant (RUQ) pain. Right sided pleural effusion is also common (in 20-30% of patients). Infection occurs primarily in tropical developing countries such as Mexico. Eosinophilia is commonly associated with parasitic infections (generally caused by helminths). Clinical diagnosis of amebic liver abscess is nonspecific and is usually confirmed by radiology to identify the abscess, followed by serology or aspiration of the abscess for microbiological studies. Differential diagnosis includes pyogenic abscess, lung or gallbladder disease, and any other febrile illness (as some patients present only with fever).

Although it is not uncommon for appendicitis to present with pain outside the usual RL abdominal quadrant, this patient does not have the typical features of acute **appendicitis** such as anorexia, nausea, and vomiting. In addition, this patient does not have typical features of acute appendicitis such as anorexia, nausea, and vomiting. **Cholecystitis** is unlikely due to no history of fatty food intolerance and negative Murphy's sign (when deep palpation under the right costal margin causes extreme pain and inhibits inspiration). **Hepatitis** may present with RUQ pain and fever, but jaundice, nausea, and vomiting might be expected as well. **Pyogenic abscess** may have a similar presentation, but is not associated with eosinophilia or travel to Mexico.

Fauci, 14th ed., pp 1164, 1170, 1176-79, 1658.

118

(Block 3: Item 18)

(B)

This patient has the classic presentation of tension pneumothorax and requires immediate **insertion of a left thoracostomy tube**. Tension pneumothorax is usually caused by blunt or penetrating trauma, and is the most common life-threatening thoracic injury. The lung integrity is compromised, allowing a connection between the pleural space and the outside air via the lung or bronchial tree. This causes an increase in pleural pressure, collapsing the lung and leading to decreased breath sounds on the ipsilateral side. Increased pressure causes the trachea to deviate to the contralateral side and impedes venous return to the heart, causing hypotension and shock. Central venous hypervolemia, caused by obstructed venous return, may result in distended neck veins. However, many of these symptoms can be absent. Lactated Ringer's solution or normal saline are typically used to correct volume depletion such as that which occurs with hemorrhage. In this case, however, the patient is not truly hypovolemic but hypotensive due to decreased venous return. Initial treatment is insertion of a thoracostomy tube on the ipsilateral side, usually in the fourth or fifth intercostal space at the midaxillary line. This decompresses the pleural space and results in clinical improvement.

Intubation is indicated in patients with decreased consciousness, hypotension, major head or neck injury, chest trauma, or cyanosis. This patient is alert and coherent and his hypotension will likely resolve if the tension pneumothorax is treated. **Infusion of type-specific un-crossmatched blood** is indicated only for hypovolemic shock; in these situations, O-negative blood can be used, if there is still shock after an initial resuscitation with about 2 L of crystalloid. Un-crossmatched blood is started immediately for obvious exsanguinating injuries; usually these patients will be going directly to the OR. Again, though this patient may progress to profound shock, he requires thoracostomy to reverse this process. **Peritoneal lavage** is used in cases of abdominal injury when it is unclear whether surgical abdominal exploration is necessary, especially when the patient is unstable. The bladder and stomach are emptied and a catheter is inserted below the umbilicus. Fluid is infused and aspirated, and assessed for blood, fecal matter, or bacteria. Presence of any of these indicates abdominal exploration. **Pericardiocentesis** is a treatment for cardiac tamponade, which results from the rapid accumulation of fluid in the pericardial sac. Increased pressure restricts venosus return and ventricular filling. Cardiac tamponade due to trauma is often fatal within minutes, but if the patient survives, the classic triad of symptoms is hypotension, distended neck veins, and muffled heart sounds.

Forrest, pp 27, 156.
Rambo, pp 222-24, 242-46.
Ritchie, pp 860-62, 866-67.

119

(Block 3: Item 19)

(B)

Chronic bronchitis is defined clinically as productive cough for over 3 months during two consecutive years. (Note that emphysema is defined pathologically by abnormally enlarged air spaces distal to the terminal bronchiole caused by a compromise in the integrity of alveolar walls and alveolar wall breakdown. Both chronic bronchitis and emphysema are part of chronic obstructive pulmonary disease or COPD.)

Pulmonary function tests in COPD classically reveal a markedly decreased FEV_1 to FVC ratio. Chronic bronchitis is usually caused by persistent irritation of the airways, typically from smoking. Hypersecretion of mucus results in airway obstruction. Moreover, smoking tends to interfere with the mucociliary escalator, predisposing to infection. The usual progression of chronic bronchitis ("blue bloater") is increased productive cough, especially in the morning, and frequent respiratory infections, particularly in the winter. If patients continue to smoke, dyspnea on exertion and cyanosis may eventually result. Other potential consequences of smoking include cor pulmonale (right ventricular hypertrophy and eventual failure due to pulmonary disease) and lung cancer. **Cessation of smoking** will minimize the chances of all of these sequelae and will improve this patient's long-term prognosis more than any other treatment.

This patient should receive **yearly influenza virus immunization** since she has chronic lung disease, though this will not offer as much benefit as smoking cessation. A **regular exercise program** will not ameliorate the lung damage, though it will improve her respiratory capacity, especially since she is sedentary. Medical treatments for COPD include the inhaled bronchodilators ipratropium and β-adrenergic agonists such as albuterol, oral and inhaled corticosteroids, and oral theophylline. Inhaled ipratropium, **β-adrenergic agonist inhalers**, and inhaled and oral steroids are principal pharmacological treatments for COPD. **Daily percussion and postural drainage** can improve pulmonary function by clearing the airways of mucus, but these treatments address the symptoms, and not the cause of the disease, and therefore have little impact on long-term prognosis.

Cotran, 6th ed., pp 688-89.
Tierney, 38th ed., pp 277-79.

120

(Block 3: Item 20)

(A)

History of colon surgery suggests infection originating from the gut. Fever with shaking chills could be caused by sepsis by any Gram-negative organism, through the actions of endotoxin. Gentamicin and ampicillin are effective antibiotics for Gram-negative bacterial infections; they do not cover anaerobes effectively. ***Bacteroides fragilis*** is an anaerobic, gram-negative bacterium found in the normal flora of the gut; it is also one of the most antibiotic-resistant of the anaerobes and produces beta-lactamase (rendering penicillins, like ampicillin, useless). *Bacteroides* is also resistant to first-generation cephalosporins and aminoglycosides (e.g., gentamicin). The drug of choice for this organism is metronidazole (Flagyl), with cefoxitin, clindamycin, chloramphenicol, β-lactam/β-lactamase inhibitors, or carbapenems as other options.

All the other bacteria listed are also Gram-negative rods. Infection with ***Brucella abortus*** is usually zoonotic (from an animal source). It is sensitive to gentamicin. Like Bacteroides, ***E. coli*** is also found in the GI tract, but it is sensitive to gentamicin (and sometimes sensitive to ampicillin as well). *E. coli* can cause sepsis and is a major cause of urinary tract infections and traveler's diarrhea. ***Proteus mirabilis*** is also a member of the normal colonic flora and can also cause both urinary tract infections as well as Gram-negative sepsis. However, it is usually sensitive to ampicillin and gentamicin. ***Pseudomonas aeruginosa*** is less frequently a member of normal colonic flora but is often found in soil or water. It is usually associated with burn wound infections, pneumonia (especially in cystic fibrosis patients), and urinary tract infections. The treatment of choice for *Pseudomonas* is usually an extended-spectrum penicillin and aminoglycoside.

Levinson, 3rd ed., pp 97-100, 107-11, 117.

121

(Block 3: Item 21)

(D)

The natural evolution of colon cancer usually begins with a benign, hyperplastic adenomatous polyp. As the polyp increases in size, so do the chances of malignant transformation. Eventually, invasive carcinoma can develop, and metastases can occur after invasion of the muscularis mucosa. Early treatment is vital, as surgical excision can be curative. Unfortunately, 25-30% of patients with colorectal carcinoma are inoperative at diagnosis due to metastatic spread. Typical presentation is an older individual with anemia or occult blood in the stool. Adenomas are often asymptomatic and discovered incidentally on routine screening by flexible sigmoidoscopy. Since this patient's polyp was found by colon contrast study, the patient should undergo **colonoscopy with polypectomy**. An abnormal contrast study is an indication for colonoscopy for two reasons: other polyps may have been missed and histologic examination of the excised polyp upon excision is necessary for diagnosis. If a screening sigmoidoscopy demonstrates a polyp, polypectomy should be done during the sigmoidoscopy and the patient should then have a colonoscopy to look for polyps in the more proximal portions of the colon. Peak incidence of colorectal carcinoma is 60-70 years. Because our patient is younger and has no family history of colon cancer, suspicion for peptic ulcer disease and, possibly, gastric carcinoma merited the upper GI series.

A **reexamination in 1 year** would miss a possible early diagnosis and thereby allow any neoplastic transformation to progress unchecked. Meat and iron in the diet can cause false positive tests for occult blood in the stool. **Repeating the test after**

3 days on a meat-free diet would be reasonable in a young patient who has a low probability of having occult bleeding but has a positive test. However, once a polyp is found, additional testing for occult blood is not helpful. Colon cancers often over-express serum carcinoembryonic antigen (CEA). However, **measurement of (CEA) level** is neither sensitive nor specific, so it is not useful as a screening test for colon cancer. The test can be useful for following the progression of cancer after surgical excision, as rising CEA levels may indicate recurrence. **Total colectomy** is overkill, as a 1.5-cm polyp is likely benign and, in any case, first requires pathologic diagnosis to establish an optimal assessment and plan.

Cotran, 5th ed., pp 809-17.
Fauci, 14th ed., p 1587.

122

(Block 3: Item 22)

(A)

This patient has **axillary-subclavian venous thrombosis**; obstruction usually occurs where the vein passes the first rib (duplex ultrasound can document this condition). Venous thrombosis causes local symptoms, such as distal edema (nonpitting), cyanosis, dilatation of superficial veins, and pain. Enlarged cutaneous veins over the chest wall indicates alternative venous drainage through superficial veins leading to the intercostal veins, then to the azygos vein which drains into the superior vena cava proximal to the thrombosis in the axillary-subclavian vein. Worsening of the pain with exercise is due to increased blood flow to the arm with limited ability to increase venous drainage through these accessory pathways, leading to exacerbation of swelling and pain. Operation of a jackhammer may predispose to development of thrombi due to mechanical disruption of blood vessels.

Deep venous valvular insufficiency of an extremity is usually a chronic post-phlebitic process manifest as edema, hyperpigmentation, and secondary superficial varicose veins. It usually occurs in the distal leg and ankle. **Superficial thrombophlebitis of the breast** could account for the enlarged chest veins but is unlikely to cause symptoms in the arm, since venous blood from the arm does not drain into superficial veins of the breast. Similarly, **superficial thrombophlebitis of the cephalic vein** would disrupt some venous drainage in the arm but would be compensated for by drainage through the basilic and brachial veins, and thus could not explain the enlarged chest veins. **Thrombosis of preexisting upper extremity varicosities** would not explain chest vein enlargement since deep venous drainage would be unaffected.

Cotran, 5th ed., pp 504-06.
Fauci, 14th ed., pp 1403-05.

123

(Block 3: Item 23)

(E)

The history suggests toxic shock syndrome (TSS), which is usually caused by *Staphylococcus aureus.* The syndrome classically occurs in tampon users (though it can also follow septic abortions, burns, or surgery). Bacteria grow in and around the tampon and then secrete a toxin (toxic shock syndrome toxin-1, TSST-1), thereby inducing toxic shock syndrome. This is a "superantigen" which binds to the T-cell receptor and activates it nonspecifically, causing massive immune system activation. The clinical picture includes abrupt onset of fever, vomiting, watery diarrhea, sore throat, myalgias, and headache; a diffuse, maculopapular erythematous rash that desquamates (especially, on the palms and soles) is classic. Hypotension with renal and cardiac failure occurs in severe cases. Since *Staphylococci* are usually resistant to penicillin, a penicillinase-resistant penicillin is required, such as **Nafcillin**. Management should also include fluid administration, correction of renal or cardiac dysfunction, and removal of the source of the toxin (i.e. remove tampon, drain abscess). Fatality rates may approach 15%.

Ampicillin is susceptible to penicillinases (β-lactamases) and therefore not a good choice for TSS. **Chloramphenicol** has potentially toxic side effects (including irreversible aplastic anemia) so is usually only used for serious infections in patients allergic to β-lactam antibiotics. **Doxycycline** and **tetracycline** are most commonly given for *Mycoplasma* and *Chlamydia* infections. **Gentamicin**, an aminoglycoside, is useful against aerobic Gram-negative bacteria such as *Pseudomonas* and *Enterobacter.*

Cotran, 5th ed., pp 335-37.
Levinson, 3rd ed., pp 73-76.
Mycek, 2nd ed., pp 297-303, 311-17, 320-21.
Tierney, 38th ed., p 1298.

124

(Block 3: Item 24)

(C)

Primary dysmenorrhea usually occurs before age 20. Nausea and vomiting at the beginning of menses are classically associated with primary dysmenorrhea. Women with primary dysmenorrhea have higher tissue levels of prostaglandins, which cause pain by either stimulating uterine contractions and cramps or by causing uterine ischemia. Prostaglandins are produced during the luteal phase, after ovulation. If no ovulation occurs, there are no prostaglandins and no cramps. Therefore, there are two main options for therapy. First is prostaglandin synthesis inhibitors. The other option is oral contraceptive pills (OCPs) to prevent ovulation. Aspirin can be used for dysmenorrhea, but it is often not efficacious. **Ibuprofen** is another non-steroidal anti-inflammatory that acts by reversibly inhibiting cyclo-oxygenase, thereby inhibiting prostaglandin synthesis from arachidonic acid. Though the mechanism is similar, indomethacin is generally better for dysmenorrhea than aspirin and causes fewer gastrointestinal side effects. OCPs can be used in patient who cannot get relief from NSAIDs or cannot tolerate them.

The other drugs are not relevant to the pathophysiology of our patient's pain. **Doxycycline**, an antibiotic, can be given for chlamydial pelvic inflammatory disease, but this patient has no signs or symptoms of infection. **Acetaminophen** is another cyclo-oxygenase inhibitor; however, its actions are concentrated in the CNS. It relieves pain centrally, but does not help prevent uterine cramps or ischemia. **Codeine**, an opioid with anti-tussive (cough suppressant) properties, also only addresses the symptom of pain, and not the underlying process. Furthermore, codeine is sedating and constipating. **Danazol** is an androgen that can be used for treating endometriosis. This patient has a classic case of dysmenorrhea, not endometriosis.

Callahan, 1st ed., p 140.
Fauci, 14th ed., p 290.
Goroll, 3rd ed., pp 614-18.
Tierney, 38th ed., pp 1533-36.

125

(Block 3: Item 25)

(E)

Neisseria gonorrhoeae infection in men typically presents with purulent urethral discharge. Gram stain and culture of the discharge confirm diagnosis. In men, Gram stain showing Gram-negative diplococci inside neutrophils is sufficient for diagnosis. In women, culture is recommended since smears are often negative. Treatment of gonococcal infection is usually with ceftriaxone; often, tetracycline is coadministered to cover mixed infection with *Chlamydia*. Although penicillin was used in this case, *N. gonorrhoeae* is penicillin-resistant (30-50% of the cases). Partners should also be tested and treated, especially because gonorrhea is often asymptomatic (especially in women) and can colonize oral and anal areas from which reinfection can occur. In this case, **reinfection from the partner** is likely; the partner's anal fissure suggests that he may be infected despite his negative urethral culture. Oral and anal infections can both be asymptomatic or cause local inflammation (pharyngitis or proctitis, with bloody or purulent discharge).

Bacterial resistance could have emerged since the original culture, if the offending bacteria acquired a plasmid conferring penicillin-resistance. However, this patient likely acquired the same bacterium from his partner, and we are told it is still penicillin-sensitive. **Inadequate treatment with penicillin** is unlikely, assuming the patient received a standard course of treatment. **Concurrent herpesvirus infection** and **alcohol intake**, which may both predispose to infection (by the presence of mucosal lesions and impaired immune response, respectively) would not interfere with proper therapy to cause persistence of infection or reinfection.

Tierney, 38th ed., pp 1319-20.

126

(Block 3: Item 26)

(C)

Polymyalgia rheumatica (PMR) is a clinical syndrome characterized by polymyalgias (pain) and polyarthralgias (stiffness) mainly of the back, shoulders, neck, and pelvic girdle muscles. Symptoms are typically worse in the morning (on awakening) and at night. PMR often coexists with temporal (giant cell) arteritis, which is a granulomatous inflammatory process, primarily of the extracranial branches of the carotid arteries. Temporal arteritis classically presents with headache, tenderness and decreased pulsation over the temporal arteries, and scalp tenderness. Both disorders occur primarily in individuals over 50 years old. In addition to pain and stiffness, patients with PMR frequently have fever, malaise, and weight loss. Depression may also be present. Aside from tenderness of the aforementioned areas, physical examination is usually unremarkable. Muscle strength is normal. Anemia is common, and a markedly elevated erythrocyte sedimentation rate (ESR) is virtually always present. The ESR is usually > 50 mm/hr, and often > 100 mm/hr. Serum creatinine kinase is normal. Some physicians recommend temporal artery biopsy in all patients with PMR because of the high incidence of associated temporal arteritis, which can lead to blindness if not promptly treated with high-dose corticosteroids. A patient with pure PMR (no symptoms or signs of temporal arteritis) can generally be treated with low-dose corticosteroids, with temporal artery biopsy reserved for those who subsequently develop symptoms of that disorder.

Hyperthyroidism can cause muscle weakness and atrophy **(hyperthyroid myopathy)**, but, rarely, muscle pain. The myopathy responds to treatment of the hyperthyroidism. In **myasthenia gravis** (MG), antibodies against the nicotinic acetylcholine receptor of the neuromuscular junction block neuromuscular transmission, resulting in muscle weakness. MG classically causes diplopia, dysphagia, and ptosis. Muscles of respiration and of the extremities may also be involved. Weakness worsens with exercise and improves with rest. The diagnosis of MG is confirmed by improvement of muscle strength in response to an anticholinesterase such as edrophonium (Tensilon). **Rheumatoid arthritis** (RA) is a systemic inflammatory disease, likely autoimmune in nature. RA primarily affects joints, not muscles, and is most common in women under age 40. Systemic symptoms include malaise, fever, and weight loss. There are many extra-articular manifestations of RA, such as subcutaneous nodules, pleural effusions, pericarditis, and vasculitis. **Steroid myopathy** (drug-induced) can present similarly to PMR with nonspecific muscle weakness and pain. However, the diagnosis is reached by taking a careful history and may be confirmed by serum tests for the steroid and its metabolites.

Cotran, 5th ed., p 1292.
Fauci, 14th ed., p 2480.
Tierney, 38th ed., pp 821-22, 985-86.

127

(Block 3: Item 27)

(A)

Inability to void is relatively common in the immediate postoperative period. Postoperative urinary retention may be caused by interference with neural mechanisms responsible for micturition and by overdistention of the bladder (> 500 mL in the bladder causes contraction rather than micturition). It can often be diagnosed and treated with **placement of a Foley catheter** in the bladder. Unless greater than 1000 mL of urine is drained, the catheter can be removed. Large volumes of intraoperative IV fluids (required after a hypotensive episode) and underlying BPH (in older men) can exacerbate acute urinary retention.

If urine output does not improve with the catheter in place, the next step is usually a **renal ultrasound**, which reveals hydronephrosis if the process is indeed due to obstruction. **CT scan of the abdomen** can be helpful if obstruction is due to tumor. The patient, in question, is slightly anemic (normal hemoglobin: 13.5-17.7 g/dL), but **transfusion of packed red blood cells** is generally reserved for more severe, symptomatic anemia. This patient is also slightly hyperglycemic. However, serum glucose of less than 200 is generally acceptable during a hospitalization and **administration of 20 U of regular insulin** could cause severe hypoglycemia.

Facui, 14th ed., pp 260, 1558-59.
Tierney, 38th ed., pp 867-69.
Way, 10th ed., p 35.

128

(Block 3: Item 28)

(E)

The confidentiality of the doctor-patient relationship can only be broken in cases where the physician finds that there is danger of harm to others. The 1974 *Tarasoff* decision provides the legal precedent for this (*Tarasoff v. Regents of CA et al.*). The case specifically addressed the requirements of physicians to notify law enforcement officials and the intended victims of a patient's threats. It was found that the containment of such risks falls within the public interest. Although the *Tarasoff* case is only legally binding in the California courts, many other states have followed this approach and have adopted the duty to warn third parties under certain circumstances. Other exceptions to doctor-patient confidentiality include: HIV-patients who habitually put other sexual partners at risk by nondisclosure; child abuse; and suicidal intent.

In this situation, no risk of harm to others is present and confidentiality cannot be breached, despite the status of the hospital administrator. The surgeon should **decline to answer, because the information is confidential**.

Jonsen, 4th ed., pp 166-73.
Hall, pp 376-84.
Tarasoff v. Regents of CA et al., 17 Cal. 3d 425; 551 (1976)

129

(Block 3: Item 29)

(D)

This infant has isolated microcytic, hypochromic anemia (hematocrit of 25%). Normal mean hematocrit for this age (6 months-2 years) is 36% with a lower limit of 33%. The most common cause of this type of anemia is iron deficiency. Despite a normal, balanced diet, iron may be deficient; during periods of growth, especially in infancy, more iron is needed than in normal adults. Breast-fed infants usually are less at risk for iron deficiency, as the iron in breast milk is more readily absorbed than iron from other dietary sources. Therefore, infants not being breast-fed should be given **iron-fortified diets** (such as **regular consumption of iron-containing formula**). Premature infants, such as this baby who was born at 33 weeks, are susceptible to anemia, since secondary iron stores are primarily established during the 3rd trimester.

Of the other nutritional deficiencies, only **vitamin C** and **E** deficiency cause hematologic symptoms. Skeletal changes, poor wound healing, and skin rash characterizes **Vitamin C** deficiency, or scurvy. Often, anemia is present as well, though it is usually normochromic and normocytic and due to bleeding into tissues. **Vitamin E deficiency** can cause a hemolytic anemia in infants, though this is most likely a normochromic, normocytic anemia. Recommended feeding for infants less than 6 months of age is breast milk or formula. Solid food is generally not recommended until 4-6 months of age; **introduction of fresh fruits and vegetables at 3 months** would be considered too early and would not correct the infant's anemia. **Regular consumption of 2% milk** only ensures fat and calorie consumption, not iron.

Cotran, 5th ed., pp 418-19, 423-25.
Nelson, 3rd ed., pp 58-63, 548-56.

130

(Block 3: Item 30)

(C)

All expectant mothers are screened for hepatitis B surface antigen (HBsAg). Those positive for HBsAg are likely to have chronic disease and pose a risk of transmission to the fetus via the placenta. Since serologic testing in this patient is also positive for IgM-anti-hepatitis B core antigen (IgM-anti-HBcAg), this mother (with hepatomegaly and plausible exposure via her husband) has been recently infected by hepatitis B. She is in the "window period," when only anti-HBcAg is detected. Moreover, the antibody is of the IgM class, indicating recent primary exposure to the antigen. Usually, hepatitis B can be detected within the first 4-5 months by the HBsAg (the surface antigen of the virus particle). Then, in the window period at about 6 months, only anti-HBcAg antibody can be detected, and afterwards anti-HBs antibody is present as well, indicating convalescence (recovery). Immunized individuals have anti-HBs, and not anti-HBc. Major modes of transmission are by blood, sexual contact, or birth (any bodily fluids, including breast milk), though transmission in the presence of intact skin or by ingestion is rare. Therefore, the infant is at risk for infection, and standard treatment is to give both **hepatitis B immune globulin (HBIG) and the hepatitis B vaccine at birth**, an example of passive-active immunization therapy (the other condition for which passive-active therapy is used is rabies).

Either treatment in isolation is less effective and therefore not recommended. All unexposed newborns are now recommended to receive Hepatitis B vaccination. Cessation of breast-feeding to eliminate further exposure from the mother may help, but infection by oral ingestion is less common and this would deprive the infant of protective IgA antibodies in the breast milk against other diseases.

Callahan, 1st ed., p 70.
Levinson, 3rd ed., pp 219-222.

131

(Block 3: Item 31)

(C)

This boy has classic hemophilia. It is difficult to distinguish clinically between coagulation **factor VIII** (Hemophilia A) and IX (Hemophilia B or "Christmas disease") deficiency, because they have the same inheritance (X-linked) and similar bleeding characteristics. These are secondary hemostasis disorders (primary disorders affect platelet plug formation; secondary disorders affect fibrin clot formation) that result in deep muscle and joint bleeding from birth (spontaneous hemarthroses), bleeding into the gastrointestinal tract, and prolonged bleeding or oozing from superficial wounds. Patients with mild hemophilia (factor VIII:C levels > 5%) bleed only after major trauma or surgery; those with moderate disease bleed after only minor trauma or surgery (factor VIII:C levels 1-5%), and those patients with severe hemophilia (factor VIII:C levels < 1%) bleed spontaneously. PTT (partial thromboplastin time) is prolonged, and all other coagulation studies (PT, bleeding time, and fibrinogen) are normal. The early onset, sex of the child, family history, and coagulation studies all affirm the diagnosis. Definitive diagnosis rests on demonstrating lowered serum factor VIII:C levels. Hemophilia is the most common and serious of the genetic disorders of the clotting cascade. It occurs because a complex of activated Factor IX and Factor VIII are required to activate Factor X in the intrinsic pathway. Factor X then activates Factor II (prothrombin) along with Factor V to activate thrombin-mediated cleavage of fibrinogen to form the clot. Treatment is based on infusion of recombinant factor VIII, though expensive. Factor VIII concentrates (heat-treated to reduce transmission of HIV) are used less frequently.

Deficiencies of clotting factors besides VIII and IX can also cause bleeding disorders, but are extremely rare. **Factor VII** deficiency is autosomal recessive and causes a normal PTT but prolonged PT, and patients have severe bleeding. **Factor X** deficiency is also autosomal recessive and causes bleeding; both PTT and PT should be prolonged. **Factor XIII** deficiency is also autosomal recessive and usually presents with umbilical stump bleeding after birth (or, later, with delayed bleeding after trauma or surgery); PTT and PT are normal. **Factor III** is now recognized as tissue factor; deficiency is not a consideration.

Babior, 3rd ed., pp 189-208.
Fauci, 14th ed., pp 736-39.
Tierney, 38th ed., pp 527-28.

132

(Block 3: Item 32)

(B)

Basal cell epithelioma (or carcinoma) commonly presents in older patients as sun-damaged areas of the head and neck. The lesions are "translucent papules with rolled borders, telangiectasias, and central erosion." They may have a waxy, pearly appearance and may ulcerate if neglected. This patient presents a classic case: he is an older man, the erythematous areas indicate sun damage, and the appearance of the lesion is typical. This is a sporadic case, though there are inherited forms (basal cell nevus syndrome) that usually present before the age of 30. Basal cell epithelioma is the most common cancer in the US. Though malignant and locally invasive, metastatic potential is very low, and these lesions are routinely cured by excision. They can recur and proper excision may produce cosmetic deformity. Sun avoidance and regular physician follow-up is recommended.

Actinic keratosis (AK) typically has a rough surface, sometimes a "cutaneous horn," and is brown, red, or skin-colored; they are considered premalignant lesions and also occur on sun-exposed areas of the skin. **Kaposi's sarcoma** (caused by human herpes virus 8) is a malignant tumor of mesenchymal cells that appear as red, purple, or dark nodules or plaques on cutaneous or mucosal surfaces. Outside of AIDS-related cases, it is very rare and tends to cluster in Eastern Europeans or Mediterraneans (classic or European form), where lesions occur on lower extremities, or in African children, where it can resemble lymphoma. **Melanoma** is an increasingly common malignancy and the leading cause of death from skin disease. Lesions are often asymptomatic, may be flat or raised, and have irregular borders and variegated coloring. The majority of melanomas occur *de novo* on the skin and are not associated with the patient's normal nevi. The most common symptom of a melanoma is pruritus (again, most are asymptomatic). Other worrisome signs of melanoma include increasing size (growing faster in proportion to the individual's growth), changing color, or spontaneous bleeding/crusting. Tumor thickness is the single most important prognostic factor. **Seborrheic keratosis** (SK) is a benign tumor of older individuals. They appear as brown, round, flat plaques with a "stuck-on" or velvety/warty appearance. Often it may be difficult to distinguish between squamous cell carcinoma, basal cell carcinoma, and benign disorders such as AK or SK. When there is doubt, a biopsy for tissue diagnosis is necessary.

Cotran, 5th ed., pp 511-12, 1179-86.
Fauci, 14th ed., p 323.
Tierney, 38th ed., pp 123-24, 129, 160-61, 163.

133

(Block 3: Item 33)

(C)

This boy shows typical symptoms (seasonal nasal discharge and watery, itchy eyes) of atopic (Type I) hypersensitivity, responsible for common allergies. A skin test with suspected antigens may verify the offending antigen. In this case, erythema and wheal reaction within 15 minutes is characteristic of Type I hypersensitivity. Type I hypersensitivity is due to IgE antibodies directed against the offending antigen. These IgE antibodies are anchored on the surface of mast cells; binding of antigen leads to dimerization of the antibodies, signaling the **mast cell to release histamine** and other inflammatory mediators that are preformed and stored in its granules. In turn, histamine increases vascular permeability and causes vasodilation, accounting for the erythema and wheal. Also, the binding of antigen to IgE antibodies causes synthesis of other inflammatory mediators such as leukotrienes and prostaglandins **(release of lymphokines from mast cells)**; they are responsible for the "late phase response"—enhanced vascular permeability, bronchial smooth muscle contraction (allergic asthma), and increased mucus secretion. The "late phase response" occurs on the time scale of hours rather than minutes.

Type II hypersensitivity occurs when antibody directed at antigens of the cell membrane activates complement, generating a membrane-attack complex and resulting in cell lysis. Examples include ABO transfusion reactions and drug-induced hemolysis or thrombocytopenia. Type III hypersensitivity is due to **circulating antibody-antigen complexes**. The complexes are deposited in tissues and result in an inflammatory response via activated complement. Examples include serum sickness and the Arthus reaction (local tissue necrosis due to immune-complex vasculitis). Type IV (delayed, cell-mediated) hypersensitivity is T cell mediated. T cells sensitized to an antigen are activated upon subsequent exposure, causing inflammation due to **activated CD4+ T cells releasing lymphokines** (IFN-gamma, IL-2, and TNF-alpha); lymphokines then **recruit phagocytes** and other inflammatory cells that cause erythema, itching, vesication, eczema, and necrosis within 12-48 hours. This is commonly seen in the tuberculin response when testing for exposure to *Mycobacterium tuberculosis.*

Cotran, 5th ed., pp 178-90.
Levinson, 3rd ed., pp 330-31.

134

(Block 3: Item 34)

(A)

The child has trisomy 21, or Down's syndrome, the most common autosomal chromosomal abnormality. The incidence of this disorder is 1 in 700 live births in the U.S. The risk of having a child with trisomy 21 increases with advancing maternal age, rising dramatically after age 35 (1 in 25 live births of mothers over 45 are affected). **Screening by amniocentesis for karyotype** at 15-17 weeks gestation is recommended for mothers aged 35 and older. Affected infants have flat faces, a flat nasal bridge with epicanthic folds, up-slanted palpebral fissures, a protruding tongue, micrognathia, gap between the first and second toes, single palmar creases, and clinodactyly (incurved fifth finger). They also can have congenital heart defects (endocardial cushion defects and septal defects in 50% of cases), duodenal atresia, Hirschsprung's disease, hypotonia, hypothyroidism, atlantoaxial instability, developmental delay, and moderate mental retardation. In addition, they are at greater risk for leukemia, Alzheimer's-like dementia (developing during 3rd and 4th decades), and infections (due to abnormal immune responses).

An **antepartum nonstress test (NST)** is a procedure that uses external monitoring to evaluate the health of the unborn baby. An external fetal monitor is attached to the mother and records the baby's heart rate; the heart rate accelerates when the baby moves. If the heart rate rises above baseline for 15 seconds twice in 20 minutes, the test is called formally reactive and the baby is considered to be healthy. NST may be indicate for mothers that are high-risk, have notice less fetal movement, or are post-dates. Trisomy 21 fetuses would have normal NSTs. Cytomegalovirus (CMV) infection during pregnancy can cause cytomegalic inclusion disease and small-for-gestational age infants. This can result in congenital abnormalities such as microcephaly, hydrocephaly, chorioretinitis, cerebral calcifications and hepatosplenomegaly. Primary infections of the mother are much more likely to be transmitted to the infant transplacentally. Though 1-2% of all infants are infected in utero, only 10% suffer clinically recognized illness. **CMV titers** may help in assessing CMV infection, but there is currently no treatment or prophylaxis for the disease. **Measurement of maternal serum alpha-fetoprotein (MSAFP) level** is performed at 15 to 19 weeks' gestation. Low values can indicate risk for Trisomy 21, but amniocentesis provides definitive diagnosis. Elevated alpha-fetoprotein levels are correlated with neural tube defects, abdominal wall defects (gastroschisis and omphalocele), multiple gestations, fetal demise, and placental abnormalities. MSAFP is usually augmented with levels of estriol and hCG ("triple screen"); Trisomy 21 babies have decreased estriol and elevated hCG in addition to decreased MSAFP. Rubella (German measles) infection in utero can cause congenital rubella syndrome; transmission from the infected mother is highest during the 1st trimester. Defects depend on the time of infection, but congenital rubella syndrome typically includes deafness, heart abnormalities, cataracts, and mental retardation (and numerous latent sequelae). The diagnosis of rubella is based on demonstrating **IgM rubella titers** in the infant since IgM does not cross the placenta. IgM titers in the mother can occur with primary and reinfection with rubella. Expectant mothers are usually checked for rubella titer during the 1st trimester; women with low or nonexistent titer should avoid possible exposure to rubella.

Callahan, 1st ed., pp 8-9, 69-70.
Marino, 1st ed., pp 95-96.
Nelson, 3rd ed., pp 145-46, 387-89, 405-06.

135

(Block 3: Item 35)

(A)

Dermatomyositis is polymyositis with characteristic skin involvement. Polymyositis refers to skeletal muscle damage due to lymphocytic inflammation. Weakness usually involves the proximal muscle groups, starting in the hips and thighs and then progressing to involve the shoulders as well. Hip and thigh weakness commonly causes difficulty rising or climbing stairs. The pattern of skin involvement in dermatomyositis consists of a purple-red (lilac-colored) rash over the upper eyelids, nose, and cheeks, sometimes in a butterfly distribution that may resemble SLE. The rash may also be found on the forehead, chest, and extensor surfaces of the extremities. Sometimes scaling occurs (heliotrope erythema). About one-third of cases have pathognomonic Gottron's papules—violaceous papules on the extensor surfaces of the hand joints, elbows, knees, or malleoli. Long-standing cases may show poikiloderma vasculare atrophicans, which is hypo- or hyperpigmentation, atrophy, and telangiectasia. Skin changes may precede or follow muscle symptoms. Polymyositis and dermatomyositis account for a majority of all cases of myositis, but the differential diagnosis for muscle weakness also includes neurological damage, neuromuscular junction defects (myasthenia gravis, Lambert-Eaton syndrome), infection (especially viral), and drug-induced myopathy. Women are affected twice as often as men, and there is no age preference. Sometimes the condition coexists with rheumatoid arthritis, SLE, mixed connective tissue disorder, progressive systemic sclerosis, or malignancy (especially when rash is present in an older individual).

Mixed connective tissue disease ("overlap connective tissue disease" or MCTD) is a disease with overlapping features of SLE, scleroderma, and polymyositis. Anti-U_1 RNP (a nuclear autoantibody) titers are usually high. MCTD may develop into one predominant disease with time. **Psoriasis** usually shows skin lesions that are pink-colored with silver-white scales. Myopathy is sometimes present in psoriasis. **Rheumatoid arthritis** is an inflammatory joint disease, and though sometimes coexistent with dermatomyositis, does not inherently affect either the skin or muscle.

Rather, weakness and limitation of motion is due to joint inflammation, and typically occurs in the distal extremities (hands, wrists, feet, and knees) instead of the proximal ones. **Systemic lupus erythematosus** (SLE) also can be associated with dermatomyositis. Multisystem involvement is usually present in SLE, so that musculoskeletal and cutaneous symptoms are accompanied by generalized symptoms (fever, malaise, weight loss) and serologic criteria (anti-dsDNA and anti-Smith antibodies), as well as a host of neurologic, pulmonary, cardiac, renal, GI, and vascular findings.

Cotran, 5th ed., pp 1197-98.
Fauci, 14th ed., pp 1872-1901.
Tierney, 38th ed., pp 817-18.

136

(Block 3: Item 36)

(D)

The differential diagnosis for an adolescent male with sudden onset of scrotal pain, swollen, erythematous scrotum, and ipsilateral absence of the cremasteric reflex should always include **torsion of the testis** and torsion of the testicular appendix or epididymis. This is a surgical emergency! Immediate operation to restore blood supply to the affected testis and prevent testicular infarction is mandatory. Complete torsion of the spermatic cord may result in testicular infarction within 4-6 hours. Classically, torsion of the testis occurs in the 10 to 20-year-old age group and presents with sudden onset of scrotal and lower abdominal pain and scrotal swelling. The exquisitely painful testis may have a "high lie" in relation to the other testis. Diagnosis can be confirmed by radionuclide perfusion scan or Doppler flow study.

Epididymitis is most commonly seen in sexually active men under 35, is associated with urethritis, and is usually caused by *Chlamydia trachomatis* (less commonly by *Neisseria gonorrhoeae*). Acute epididymitis features fever, scrotal swelling, pain in the scrotal that may radiate along the spermatic cord or to the flank, and associated symptoms of urethritis or cystitis. Prehn's sign (elevation of the scrotum improves pain from epididymitis) may help in establishing the diagnosis. **Hemorrhagic tumors** would most likely be preceded by asymptomatic testicular enlargement. Occasionally, patients may have spontaneous bleeding into the tumor mass that causes pain. Transillumination or scrotal ultrasound may be helpful. **Incarcerated hernias** in the scrotum may cause scrotal pain that can be difficult to distinguish from testicular pain. Bowel sounds may be heard in the scrotum early in the incarceration, but may disappear if the hernia strangulates. Intestinal hernia in the scrotum almost always features clinical findings of bowel obstruction. Ultrasound can aid in the diagnosis. **Torsion of the testicular appendix** can present in a similar fashion to torsion of the testicle, though it would not be expected to cause swelling and elevation of the entire testicle in the early stage. Occasionally, palpation of a small mass on the superior pole of the testis is possible, and it may give a classic "blue dot sign" when the skin is stretched over it.

Cotran, 6th ed., pp 1014-15, 1020-21.
Fauci, 14th ed., pp 804, 1057.
Goroll, pp 379-80.
Ritchie, p 523.
Tierney, 38th ed., pp 881, 905-06.
Way, 10th ed., pp 959-60.

---

137 & 138

(Block 3: Items 37 & 38)

(A) & (A)

respectively

This patient has **hypercalcemia** of malignancy and should be treated **with intravenous bisphosphonate** (pamidronate). Hypercalcemia of malignancy is the most common paraneoplastic syndrome and accounts for 40% of all cases of hypercalcemia. Circulating parathyroid hormone related peptide (PTHrP) usually causes "humoral hypercalcemia of malignancy" (HHM). HHM mimics hyperparathyroidism, causing bone absorption, increased renal absorption of calcium, and phosphaturia. Symptoms of hypercalcemia include malaise, fatigue, confusion, polyuria, polydipsia, constipation, nausea, and vomiting. Common tumors associated with HHM are non-small cell lung cancer (e.g., squamous cell carcinoma), breast cancer, renal cell carcinoma, bladder cancer, and various head and neck cancers. The narrowed QT interval on ECG reflects increased cardiac contractility due to elevated calcium, and deadly arrhythmias may occur. Treatment of hypercalcemia consists of IV hydration with normal saline (Ringer's solution contains calcium!), furosemide (to avoid intravascular overload and enhance urinary Ca^{2+} excretion), and pamidronate (a bisphosphonate that inhibits osteoclast bone absorption). In tumor-induced hypercalcemia, pamidronate normalizes plasma calcium between 3 to 7 days following the initiation of treatment irrespective of the type of malignancy or presence of detectable metastases. This effect is dependent on initial calcium levels. Pamidronate improves symptoms associated with hypercalcemia, e.g., anorexia, nausea, vomiting and diminished mental status.

HHM has a median survival of only 1-3 months. Another form of hypercalcemia caused by local paracrine release of hormones, instead of circulating PTHrP, is called local osteolytic hypercalcemia (LOH). LOH is common in breast cancer, myeloma, lymphoma, and leukemia. LOH can be treated with **glucocorticoids** that are thought to inhibit production of the paracrine hormones. Plicamycin

(mithramycin), an anticancer drug that inhibits transcription, is specific for osteoclasts, thus inhibiting bone resorption and helping correct hypercalcemia. Mithramycin is used for malignant hypercalcemia and, less commonly, for chronic myelogenous leukemia and testicular cancer. Mithramycin, as an antineoplastic drug, has many side effects that limit its usefulness as a first-line agent for hypercalcemia; more common side effects include diarrhea, irritation or soreness of mouth, loss of appetite, and nausea and vomiting. Oral **hydrochlorothiazide**, a diuretic, would be contraindicated because it increases Ca^{2+} reabsorption by the kidney, worsening the hypercalcemia. **Mannitol**, on the other hand, a simple osmotic diuretic, will not greatly enhance the excretion of calcium, so it is less useful in management.

Chronic renal failure, hypoparathyroidism, and vitamin D deficiency can cause **hypocalcemia**. When chronic, it usually presents with muscle spasms and convulsions, mental changes (irritability, depression, and psychosis), and prolonged QT interval on ECG. **Hyperkalemia** can be due to renal failure, hypoaldosteronism, or drugs such as cyclosporine, among other causes. Symptoms include weakness, which may progress to flaccid paralysis and respiratory distress. Most important is cardiac toxicity, which can cause T-wave changes (remember the peaked T-waves), increased ECG intervals, and result in ventricular fibrillation or asystole. **Hypokalemia** can be secondary to decreased potassium intake, acid-base disorders, hormonal disorders, diarrhea, or renal disorders. Symptoms usually only occur if hypokalemia is severe (< 3 mmol/L), and can include myalgia, weakness, paralysis, and various ECG changes which can eventually lead to ventricular arrhythmias. **Hyperphosphatemia** has many potential causes, including hypoparathyroidism, acid-base disorders, tumor lysis syndrome, and excess phosphate ingestion. The most dangerous sequela is metastatic calcification, or deposition of calcium salts (mostly phosphate salts) in various tissues such as blood vessels, kidneys, lungs, and gastric mucosa. This complication can result in kidney or lung damage. **Hypophosphatemia** also has various etiologies, such as decreased intake, hyperparathyroidism, and hormonal imbalances. Symptoms include rhabdomyolysis (often seen in alcoholics during withdrawal), cardiomyopathy (reduced cardiac output and hypotension), respiratory insufficiency, skeletal demineralization, metabolic acidosis (especially when secondary to vitamin D deficiency), and nervous system dysfunction.

Fauci, 14th ed., pp 272-77, 618-19, 2241-47, 2259-63.
Mycek, 2nd ed., p 387.

139

(Block 3: Item 39)

(G)

Folic acid deficiency is the most likely cause of anemia in a patient who has not consumed fresh vegetables for 1 year. The most common cause of folate deficiency is inadequate intake—alcoholics, anorexic patients, people who do not consume fresh fruits and vegetables, and people who overcook their food. Folate is absorbed throughout the entire GI tract. Folate is an essential dietary vitamin that is required for DNA synthesis in erythropoiesis and its deficiency leads to megaloblastic anemia. Humans require 50 to 200 mcg of folic acid daily. Total body stores are approximately 5000 μg; these stores last about 2-3 months without added intake. The richest source of folic acid is green leafy vegetables and citrus fruits. It is also important to know that boiling or frying of vegetables for 5 to 10 minutes will result in destruction of nearly all of the folate content. Patients with folate deficiency may have severe megaloblastic anemia; hematocrits may be as low as 10-15%. Patients may also exhibit glossitis and have diarrhea and anorexia. Red blood cell folate level is more reliable than serum folate; < 150 ng/mL is diagnostic. Folate deficiency is treated with folic acid, 1 mg/d orally. One must be careful to not miss coexistent B_{12} deficiency. Administration of folic acid to these patients may correct the hematologic abnormalities of B_{12} deficiency, but ongoing **vitamin B_{12} deficiency** will allow neurologic damage (specifically, of spinal posterior columns—decreased vibration and position sense) to progress. In contrast to diets devoid of fresh fruits and vegetables, both iron and vitamin B_{12} deficiency are associated with vegetarian diets. Animal products are the primary source of dietary Vitamin $B_{12.}$ Animal products are also a rich source of heme iron (myoglobin and hemoglobin). Although vegetables contain non-heme iron, only 1-2% of non-heme iron is absorbed as compared to 25% of heme iron.

Iron deficiency anemia is almost always caused by bleeding in adults; serum ferritin < 12 μg/L and microcytic, hypochromic erythrocytes are typical features of iron deficiency anemia. **Anemia of chronic disease**, like iron deficiency anemia, features a microcytic, hypochromic anemia secondary to chronic, systemic inflammation or infection, cancer and liver disease. Unlike iron deficiency anemia, TIBC (total iron-binding capacity) is low in ACD, serum ferritin is normal or increased in ACD, and hematocrit rarely drops below 25%. In contrast to iron deficiency anemia, **sideroblastic anemia** features adequate iron stores in the bone marrow (remember, ringed sideroblasts); the failure in hemoglobin synthesis results from a failure to incorporate heme into protoporphyrin to form hemoglobin. Often it may represent a stage in myelodysplasia that may evolve into acute leukemia. Chronic alcohol abuse, drug toxicity, and lead poisoning can also cause sideroblastic anemia. **Autoimmune hemolytic anemia** is an acquired anemia that can rapidly cause severe anemia. It occurs when an IgG autoantibody (usually the antigen is Rh factor) is synthesized that binds to the RBC membrane. These antibody-coated RBCs are either trapped in the reticuloendothelial system (leading to splenomegaly, jaundice, and anemia) or "sheared" by splenic macrophages to form spherocytes. Patients with autoimmune hemolysis will have a positive direct Coombs test and spherocytes and a reticulocytosis on peripheral smear. **Aplastic anemia** can be caused by numerous factors that result in bone marrow failure. This results in pancytopenia and hypocellular marrow (no reticulocytosis). **Acute lymphocytic leukemia (ALL)** and **acute myelogenous leukemia (AML)** are malignancies of hematopoietic progenitor cells; monoclonal expansion of a specific cell line replaces normal bone marrow components. Pancytopenia may cause fatigue, fever, easy bruising and bleeding, and infection. Organ infiltration by leukemic cells may also occur. Some patients need medical attention for gum hypertrophy and muscle and joint pain; hyperleukocytosis can lead to "sludging" in the circulation and manifest as headache, confusion and dyspnea. **Acute blood loss** may cause hypovolemia and shock.

Fauci, 14th ed., pp 482-83.
Tierney, 38th ed., pp 485-510.

140

(Block 3: Item 40)

(I)

Sickle cell-thalassemia is a milder disease than homozygous sickle cell anemia. Reduced hemoglobin concentration in the "sickle-thal" erythrocyte leads to a slower rate of sickling. Painful crises can occur in sickle cell-thalassemia when affected individuals are exposed to hypoxic environments (i.e. exercising at high altitudes). RBC sickling is dependent on increased concentration of hemoglobin (Hgb S), hypoxia (high altitude), decreased extracellular pH (anaerobic exercise), increased extracellular osmolarity (dehydration), and decreased concentration of Hgb F. Low oxygen environments induce Hgb S polymerization and subsequent distortion of RBC morphology, changes in viscosity, sludging, ischemia, and, ultimately, organ infarction. Initiation of vascular occlusion occurs most often at the precapillary arteriolar level. Reversibly sickled cells (RSCs) have normal shape and viscosity when oxygenated. Vaso-occlusive events may be secondary to RSCs which slip into the microvasculature while oxygenated then become distorted and viscous as they become deoxygenated in vessel. Resultant increase in hypoxia and acidosis secondary to ischemia cause sickling, starting vicious cycle with an end result of organ damage. Painful crises can last hours to days and often include pain in the back, long bones, and chest. Sickle cell-thalassemia patients in 'crisis' are febrile, anemic with a reticulocytosis of 10%-25%, and may have a leukocytosis up to 25,000/mm^3.

Patients with **β-thalassemia minor** (heterozygotes for a gene resulting in either absent or reduced globin chain expression) have a modest anemia with hematocrit falling between 28% and 40%. Peripheral blood smear shows microcytic (MCV 55-75 fL), hypochromia, target cells, and basophilic stippling. RBC counts are either normal or increased.

Tierney, 38th ed., pp 485-510.

141

(Block 3: Item 41)

(A)

Acute pericarditis classically presents with severe chest pain, a precordial friction rub, and J-point elevation on ECG. Pericarditis is most commonly caused by viral infections following an upper respiratory infection (URI). Common viral etiologies include coxsackievirus A and B, echovirus, adenovirus, EBV, influenza, varicella, hepatitis, mumps, and HIV. Other causes include bacterial and fungal infections, rheumatological disorders, uremia, acute MI, post-MI (Dressler's syndrome), neoplasia, and trauma. Among the clinical features of pericarditis, precordial friction rub is the most important sign and is usually best heard at the left lower sternal border. Although severe chest pain usually presents with acute infectious pericarditis, it is often absent when the etiology is slowly developing, as in TB, cancer, or uremia. When present, chest pain is pleuritic (sharp localized pain made worse by a cough, sneeze, or deep breath), retrosternal, left precordial, and radiates to the neck, shoulder, back (trapezius ridge), arms, and epigastrium. Sitting up and leaning forward relieves the chest pain. ECG changes in acute pericarditis are due to subepicardial inflammation and usually show diffuse ST elevation in limb leads and V2 to V6 and reciprocal depressions in aVR and V1; later in the course of the disease, leads showing ST-segment elevation evolve to T-wave inversion only. Echocardiography may be used to detect and determine the amount of pericardial effusion. Treatment is symptomatic, usually with NSAIDs, but steroids are used when patients are unresponsive to NSAIDs or in severe cases.

A complication of acute pericarditis is **chronic constrictive pericardiopathy**. Fibrous scarring and adhesions between the two pericardial layers prevent the ventricles from adequately filling during diastole; this constrictive disease process causes increased venous pressures (hepatomegaly, JVD, pedal edema, ascites), decreased stroke volume, and eventually heart failure. **Myocarditis**, inflammation of the myocardium, may present with fatigue, palpitations, dyspnea, precordial discomfort, and myalgias. It usually has an infectious etiology and may evolve into sudden heart failure days to weeks after an acute febrile illness or a respiratory infection. Patients with myocarditis commonly have pleuritic chest pain along with other features of heart failure. **Pericardial tamponade** or **hemopericardium** is bleeding into the pericardium as a result of cardiac rupture (i.e. from trauma, post-MI, or postoperative complications). The patient may have tachycardia, hypotension, low pulse pressure, distended neck veins, and a paradoxical pulse. It often requires emergent pericardiocentesis. **Mitral valve disease** includes mitral valve prolapse, mitral stenosis, and mitral regurgitation; mitral valve disease, broadly speaking, may cause symptoms of left ventricular compromise—fatigue, dyspnea, orthopnea, pulmonary edema, and hemoptysis. **Rheumatic fever** may involve the mitral valve and other valves acutely, and, rarely, may lead to heart failure. **Cardiogenic shock** is a shock syndrome that results from compromised cardiac function—arrhythmias, valvular disease or pericardial disease, and "pump failure." Hallmarks of cardiogenic shock are hypotension, increased peripheral vascular resistance, inadequate organ perfusion and tachycardia. **Pleuritis** is pain due to acute inflammation of parietal pleura; pleuritic pain is localized, sharp, fleeting and worsens from cough, sneezing, or deep breathing. There are numerous causes of pleuritis and the setting in which pleuritic pain evolves helps to define the differential.

Fauci, 14th ed., pp 1334-39.
Ferri, 3rd ed., pp 202-03.
Tierney, 38th ed., pp 326, 380-81, 417-18.

142

(Block 3: Item 42)

(H)

Sudden onset of chest pain, dyspnea, cough, tachypnea, and anxiety are suggestive of a **pulmonary embolism** (PE). An accentuated pulmonary S_2 secondary to elevated pulmonary vascular pressures, and hypoxemia with a significant alveolar-arteriolar O_2 difference, suggestive of a ventilation-perfusion (V/Q) mismatch, further confirm the diagnosis of PE. More than 90% of PEs originate from deep venous thrombi (DVT) in the thigh or pelvis. Other sources of PE include tumor and infective emboli, amniotic fluid, fat, and air bubbles. Risk factors for DVT include venous stasis, endothelial injury, and hypercoagulability. Surgery is a risk factor for hypercoagulability and also causes venous stasis because of prolonged bed rest and inactivity. Malignancy is also an important risk factor for hypercoagulability. In Trousseau's syndrome, which most commonly occurs in conjunction with gastrointestinal tumors, it is thought that the release of procoagulants by tumor cells leads to activation of clotting cascade, thus increasing the risk for thrombosis. There are no pathognomonic chest X-ray findings for PE even though pulmonary infiltrates and small unilateral pleural effusion may be present (Hampton's hump). Although many patients with PE have normal ECGs, sinus tachycardia and nonspecific ST-T-wave changes are the most common findings. The classic S1Q3T3 pattern (wide S-wave in lead I, large Q-wave and inverted T-wave in lead III) may be appreciated. Arterial blood gas shows hypoxemia. Pulmonary angiography is the definitive test for diagnosis of pulmonary embolism. It is most useful when the clinical suspicion of pulmonary embolism differs significantly from the results of a ventilation/perfusion (V/Q) scan, and when the V/Q scan is of intermediate probability.

Spontaneous pneumothorax is the accumulation of air in the pleural space as a result of rupture of subpleural blebs. It is most common in tall thin men in their 2nd and 3rd decades of life. It classically presents with a sudden onset of dyspnea and ipsilateral chest pain, decreased breath sounds, diminished tactile fremitus, and hyperresonance. The extent of its clinical symptoms and signs depends on the size of the pneumothorax. Unlike PE, the chest X-ray finding of visceral pleural line is diagnostic for pneumothorax.

Fauci, 14th ed., pp 1469-70.

143

(Block 3: Item 43)

(J)

While therapeutic lithium levels are commonly associated with fine resting tremor of the hands and ataxia, toxic levels (serum levels > 2mmol/L) can lead to irreversible neurotoxicity and, rarely, cardiovascular and renal failure. Neurotoxicity involves alteration of higher cortical functions and can present as memory loss, seizures, altered motor skills, dysarthria, coma, and even death. Increased intake or decreased excretion of lithium, decreased volume of distribution (dehydration), or increased individual sensitivity to lithium can cause **lithium (medication) toxicity**. The kidney normally excretes lithium salts. Within the renal tubules there is a competitive interaction between positive cations (sodium and lithium) such that decreased tubular sodium concentrations lead to increased lithium reabsorption. Patients with low serum sodium states (those on chronic diuretics and those on salt restricted diets) are at greatest risk for developing lithium intoxication. Treatment of lithium toxicity depends on the degree of toxicity. Mild to moderate toxicity can be managed by stopping lithium intake, correcting dehydration, and maintaining appropriate fluid volume and electrolyte balance. Severe lithium toxicity requires hemodialysis in order to remove the lithium from the serum. Because it may take days before serum lithium levels are back to normal, toxicity symptoms may persist for some time.

Depressive episodes in bipolar disorder cycle with shorter manic episodes; patients that complete 4 or more cycles in 1 year without remission are termed "rapid cyclers." Lithium and valproic acid (preferred in rapid cyclers) are mood stabilizers and essential to decreasing the recurrence of mania and depressive episodes in bipolar disorder. This patient is not experiencing significant mood symptoms, but is having cognitive and neurologic symptoms.

Alcohol withdrawal would present with some similar symptoms (tremor, tachycardia, increased respiratory rate, generalized anxiety, and GI distress), however, symptoms would usually begin 5-10 hours after decreasing alcohol intake, peak in intensity on day 2 to 3, and improve by day 4 or 5. Also patients suffering from withdrawal might appear confused, ataxic, might experience delirium tremens or associated seizures, and would probably show physical signs of chronic alcoholism. An **alcohol-induced "blackout"** usually occurs at blood levels above 400 mg/dL. **Apathetic hyperthyroidism** refers to hyperthyroid disorders that present with atypical findings such as depression and lethargy. It is most common in the elderly. **Residual schizophrenia** is a form of schizophrenia that no longer features any of the prominent psychotic symptoms found in the initial disease. There are some remaining symptoms of the disorder such as eccentric behavior, emotional blunting, illogical thinking, or social withdrawal. Disturbances in appetite and sleep are sometimes signs of **masked depression**. **Generalized anxiety disorder** is the most common anxiety disorder, usually occurring at age 20-35 years with a slight predominance in women. The patient presents with disabling apprehension, anxiety, worry, irritability, hypervigilance, insomnia, and somatic complaints for at least one month. **Dementia** is unlikely because it tends to have a slow, gradual progression, rather than the acute change in cognitive function demonstrated by this patient.

Kaplan, p 2028.
Tierney, 38th ed., pp 1017, 1034.

144

(Block 3: Item 44)

(G)

Alzheimer's disease (AD) is the number one cause of dementia, accounting for 60-70% of "old-age dementia" in America. AD is a progressive disease, which starts insidiously and may take several years before its symptoms are noticed. Clinically, AD is characterized by memory loss (short term followed by long term) and impairment of at least one other cognitive function—visual spatial skills, abstract thinking, judgement, personality, behavior, language, and social functioning. Diagnosis of AD is based on clinical judgement; definitive diagnosis can only be made by microscopic examination of brain tissue (demonstrating neurofibrillary tangles, senile plaques, and amyloid angiopathy) – usually after death. Although there is no diagnostic test for AD, laboratory and imaging studies can be utilized to rule out other causes of dementia.

Diagnosis of AD is further complicated by the fact that 33% of dementias are mixtures of AD and **multi-infarct dementia**. The latter, also known as vascular dementia, is the second most common cause of dementia and accounts for about 10-20% of all dementia in the US. It is associated with hypertension and caused by decreased cerebral blood flow due to atherosclerosis and infarction of small cerebral arteries. Unlike AD, multi-infarct dementia may have a sudden onset, the progression is stepwise, and the course tends to fluctuate. Less common causes of dementia include **Pick's disease** and Korsakoff's syndrome (alcohol-related). Although AD and Pick's disease are similar in clinical course and age of onset, Pick's disease affects the personality to a greater extent. Imaging studies demonstrate lobar atrophy of the brain (particularly frontal-temporal regions) in Pick's patients whereas general atrophy as seen in AD brains. **Normal pressure hydrocephalus** (also called hydrocephalus ex-vacuo) may cause mild dementia, gait disturbance, and urinary incontinence in older patients (3 w's: wet, weird, and wobbly) and must be differentiated from AD; it occurs as parenchymal brain atrophy causes the subsequent enlargement of the ventricular spaces. **Alcohol-related dementia** is part of chronic alcoholic brain syndrome; patients can have erratic behavior, memory and recall problems. **Pseudodementia** is an old term applied to dementia in patients with depressive disorders. In the past it was thought that these patients only appeared demented and thus were given the diagnosis of pseudodementia. However, today it is theorized that the dementia is legitimate and the term "dementia syndrome of depression" is more appropriate. **Normal age-associated memory decline** does not usually impair daily function or progress like AD. **Delirium** is an acute confusional state in which consciousness (awareness) is impaired. It is frequently contrasted with dementia, which has a chronic onset and is characterized by diminished mental function (particularly diminished memory). Delirium has an extensive differential diagnosis including: drugs—anticholinergics, narcotics, and steroids; systemic problems—infection and hypoxemia; metabolic disorders—liver failure, hypoglycemia and hyperglycemia; and electrolyte imbalances—hyponatremia, hypernatremia, hypocalcemia, and hypercalcemia. **Parkinson's disease** is a chronic neurodegenerative disease distinguished by tremor, rigidity, bradykinesia, and postural instability; mild dementia may also occur.

Kaplan, 7th ed., pp 2562-65.
Tierney, 38th ed., p 534.

145

(Block 3: Item 45)

(A)

Dysphagia, or difficulty in swallowing, can result from difficulty in transferring food from the oropharynx to the esophagus (oropharyngeal dysphagia), or from impaired food transport within the esophagus (esophageal dysphagia). In esophageal dysphagia, obstructive lesions initially cause problems only with solid foods, while liquids are only affected if the lumen becomes extremely narrowed. In contrast, motility disorders (due to motor dysfunction) cause dysphagia with both liquids and solids. Although many diseases can present with dysphagia, only **achalasia** shows a dilated distal esophagus with loss of peristalsis in the distal two-thirds on barium swallow. Achalasia is a progressive idiopathic motility disorder characterized by failure of the lower esophageal sphincter (LES) to relax, increased resting tone of LES, and loss of peristalsis in the distal two-thirds of the esophagus. The pathogenesis of achalasia is thought to involve the loss of ganglionic cells leading to denervation of the esophagus. Achalasia usually presents with difficulty swallowing solids and liquids and regurgitation of undigested food. The most serious secondary complication of achalasia is the development of squamous cell carcinoma of esophagus.

Diffuse esophageal spasm (DES) is another motility disorder associated with dysphagia for solids and liquids. Unlike achalasia, it is intermittent and nonprogressive. In DES, barium swallow shows simultaneous contractions of the entire esophagus with the appearance of "corkscrews" or "rosary beads". With **esophageal cancer**, there is usually a history of smoking, alcohol use, achalasia, or Barrett's esophagus. Esophageal webs can be asymptomatic or present with intermittent, nonprogressive dysphagia for solid foods. Esophageal webs, also known as mucosal rings, are thin membranes of squamous mucosa that cause esophageal constrictions. Upper esophageal webs in association with anemia of iron deficiency are better known as **Plummer-Vinson syndrome**. **Lower esophageal webs**, also known as lower esophageal rings or Schatzki's rings, are associated with hiatal hernias. Other causes for dysphagia due to esophageal strictures include esophageal injury as with **gastroesophageal reflux disease (GERD)**, **scleroderma**, radiation, and caustic injury. They involve progressive dysphagia first to solids and later to liquids. **Peptic stricture of the esophagus** is a complication of GERD; it begins with gradual dysphagia for solid foods that progresses over months to years. Often strictures are at the gastroesophageal junction and reduce heartburn because there is a barrier to reflux. Although barium swallow is done first to evaluate the nature of dysphagia, endoscopy with biopsy must be done to differentiate strictures from webs and malignant causes.

Oropharyngeal dysphagia typically causes coughing, choking, and regurgitation immediately after swallowing. **Pharyngoesophageal (Zenker's) diverticulum** is an outpouching of pharyngeal mucosa; progressive dysphagia with regurgitation of undigested food develops over years. In contrast to a sliding hiatal hernia wherein the esophagogastric junction migrates into the thorax, in the **paraesophageal hernia** the esophagogastric junction is located in its normal position within the abdomen. The fundus of the stomach squeezes through an enlarged esophageal hiatus into the thorax. Consequently, a portion of the stomach lies within the chest alongside the esophagus. With large paraesophageal hernias, the entire stomach can protrude into the chest, often assuming an upside-down configuration. Twisting (volvulus) of the stomach or progression of the herniation can obstruct the esophagus, the stomach, or its blood supply. With a sufficient degree of volvulus, acute vascular compromise can occur with catastrophic results including gastric infarction and perforation. In **pseudobulbar palsy**, although the cranial nerves and their nuclei are intact, the loss of coordination of pharyngeal muscles results in regurgitation of food upon swallowing. Pain upon swallowing (odynophagia) is commonly due to erosive disease such as infectious esophagitis due to **candida, herpes** virus, or cytomegalovirus. These occur most commonly in immunocompromised patients. **Globus hystericus** is the sensation of having some kind of mass or lump in the throat. It sometimes occurs in depression. To a depressed individual for whom eating is a struggle, the feeling that something is stuck in the gullet can falsely appear to be a justified reason for the eating difficulty.

Fauci, 14th ed., pp 228-30, 658-59, 1590-92.
Tierney, 38th ed., pp 563-74.

146

(Block 3: Item 46)

(C)

Esophageal cancer classically presents with painful swallowing (odynophagia), progressive solid food dysphagia, and weight loss over several months. Chronic smoking and alcohol use are important risk factors for esophageal (squamous cell) cancer. Achalasia, tylosis (a genetic disease with hyperkeratosis of the palms and soles), caustic strictures of the esophagus, and other head and neck cancers are also risk factors for esophageal cancer. It is more common in men (3:1) and usually develops in individuals between 50 to 70 years of age. About half of the cancers originate in the distal one third of the esophagus. Local tumor extension into the tracheobronchial tree may form a **tracheoesophageal fistula** that may cause coughing on swallowing or pneumonia. Extension of the tumor within the mediastinum may cause chest or back pain; as with lung cancer, recurrent laryngeal involvement may produce hoarseness. Cervical or supraclavicular lymphadenopathy or hepatomegaly heralds metastatic spread. Laboratory findings commonly show anemia due to either chronic disease or occult blood loss. Although barium swallow may show narrowing of the esophagus (lesions may also appear polypoid, ulcerative, or infiltrative), endoscopic biopsy must be done to differentiate malignant from benign causes of strictures. The overall 5-year survival rate of esophageal cancer is less than 15%; most patients present with advanced disease, and surgical resection alone is mostly inadequate.

Adenocarcinoma of the esophagus is increasingly common. It occurs most often in Caucasians and in patients with Barrett's metaplasia secondary to gastroesophageal reflux. Most adenocarcinomas arise in the distal third of the esophagus.

Fauci, 14th ed., pp 688-89.
Tierney, 38th ed., pp 575-76.

147

(Block 3: Item 47)

(O)

Progressive difficulty in swallowing solids and liquids in association with Raynaud's phenomenon (fingers changing color when exposed to cold), and sclerodactyly (tightness of skin over the hands) is suggestive of **systemic scleroderma**. Other abnormalities associated with systemic scleroderma include telangiectasia, hyper- and hypopigmentation of skin, GI dysmotility, pulmonary fibrosis, and cardiac and renal failure. Of note, 80% of patients with systemic scleroderma have limited disease, frequently with the findings of CREST syndrome (calcinosis cutis [deposits of calcium in the skin in the form of nodules or plaques], Raynaud's phenomenon, esophageal involvement, sclerodactyly, and telangiectasia). Patients with CREST syndrome have an overall better prognosis. Symptoms appear in the 3rd to 5th decade; women are affected 2-3 times as frequently as men. In systemic scleroderma, progressive atrophy and fibrosis of muscularis layer of gastrointestinal tract, especially in the esophagus, results in loss of lower esophageal sphincter (LES) tone with free reflux and poor peristalsis. Dysphagia in scleroderma may be due to impaired peristalsis or may be due to peptic stricture as a result of acid reflux. Barium swallow usually shows loss of peristalsis in a dilated distal esophagus and nonfunctional lower esophageal sphincter. Localized scleroderma (morphea, linear scleroderma) does not have visceral organ involvement.

Polymyositis is a systemic inflammatory disease leading to symmetric weakness of proximal muscles. Although it does not cause dysphagia, it can occur in association with scleroderma.

Fauci, 14th ed., p 1592.
Tierney, 38th ed., pp 815-16.

148

(Block 3: Item 48)

(B, C, F, G)

Acute fever of 41°C in a 1-year-old child who is otherwise asymptomatic is suggestive of an infection and warrants a search for its source. ("Fever without focus" is defined as a febrile child, less than 3 years of age, with no focal infection found on physical exam.) Initial diagnostic studies for a fever of unknown source include **complete blood count (CBC), blood culture, urinalysis (UA), and urine culture**. CBC is always done because it may provide some clues as to the type and severity of the infection. In general, the higher the WBC or the higher the absolute neutrophil count, the greater the likelihood of bacteremia. When WBC > 15,000/mm^3, the probability increases fivefold. Recent studies have shown that 3-5% of febrile children between 3-36 months of age have occult bacteremia. Because of dangerous complications associated with invasive bacterial disease (meningitis, septic arthritis, and bacterial sepsis) it is important to do blood cultures in all children (aged 3–36 months) with fever greater than 38.5°C. Because of the nonspecific nature of symptoms of UTI, it would also important to do a urinalysis (UA) and urine culture in a 1-year-old girl with a fever of 41°C. Males < 6 months of age and females < 2 years of age with fever > 39 °C should have a urine specimen for culture collected either by catheter or suprapubic tap. Urine culture is done in addition to the UA because about 20% of children with a UTI will have a normal UA.

All other studies are done only when there are abnormal signs or symptoms suggestive of a disease. Chest X-rays and stool cultures are only performed if indicated by history or physical examination in febrile children aged 3 months - 3 years. The exception to this rule is **CSF analysis and culture** for infants less than 12 months of age and chest X-rays for febrile newborns under 4 weeks of age. Because signs and symptoms of CNS infection may be difficult to recognize in infants, CSF analysis and culture must also be done to rule out CNS infection. **Electrolyte status** is not a priority if there is no clinical suspicion of dehydration (tachycardia, oliguria, prolonged capillary refill, dry mucous membranes, "tenting" of skin, depressed fontanel).

Marino, 1st ed., pp 131-32.
Merenstein, 18th ed., pp 46-47.

149

(Block 3: Item 49)

(A, B, C, F, G, I)

Acute onset of fever of 39°C, in an asymptomatic newborn, warrants **CSF analysis and culture, blood culture, CBC, UA, and urine culture** as explained in the previous question. Most experts maintain that febrile newborns under 4 weeks of age should have a work-up for sepsis (which includes the **chest X-ray**) and be hospitalized. They are either observed or placed on parenteral antibiotics pending culture results.

A **stool culture** would only be taken if they were abnormal. **Abdominal X-ray** should only be taken if the infant is symptomatic. Since there is no suspicion of dehydration, measurement of **serum electrolyte levels** is unnecessary.

Merenstein, 18th ed., pp 46-47.

150

(Block 3: Item 50)

(B, C, I)

In children with sickle cell disease (SSD), acute fever (39.5°C) and chest pain with an abnormal chest exam warrant a **blood culture, CBC, and a chest X-ray**. Both pulmonary infection and vaso-occlusive crises can present with fever and focal tenderness. Particularly worrisome, in children with sickle cell disease (SSD), is acute chest syndrome (ACS). ACS can be defined as (1) a *new* infiltrate on chest X-ray and (2) is associated with one or more new symptoms: fever, cough, sputum production, dyspnea, or hypoxia. It is unclear if ACS is infectious or non-infectious in origin. The symptom complex may be varied, and not all symptoms are present in every episode; however, some combination of these symptoms is required for diagnosis. ACS is a common complication of the sickling disorders (Hgb SS, Hgb SC, Hgb S β^{+}-thalassemia, Hgb S β^{0}-thalassemia, etc.) and is responsible for considerable morbidity and mortality in these patients.

Children with SSD are at risk for bacteremia and their secondary complications. These patients undergo "autosplenectomy" by about 6 years of age and lose their splenic function. Autosplenectomy makes them more susceptible to bacteremia with encapsulated organisms. Therefore, it is important to do a blood culture in all febrile SSD patients to identify those at risk for development of pneumonia, meningitis, or osteomyelitis. Although some SSD patients have a baseline leukocytosis, a CBC with a left shift may help in supporting a picture of infection over infarction. Likewise, chest X-ray findings may help rule in infection over infarction.

Merenstein, 18th ed., pp 46-47.
http://www-rics.bwh.harvard.edu/sickle/acutechest.html

Bibliography

Aminoff, M., et al. *Clinical Neurology,* 3/e, Appleton and Lange, Stamford, CT, 1995.

Babior, Bernard M. and Thomas P. Stossel. *Hematology: A Pathophysiological Approach,* 3/e, Churchill Livingstone, New York, 1994.

Behrman, Ricard, Robert Kliegman, Ann Arvin, and Waldo Nelson. *Nelson's Textbook of Pediatrics,* 15/e, W. B. Saunders Co., Philadelphia, 1995.

Benson, Michael D. *Gynecologic Pearls: A Practical Guide for the Efficient Resident,* 1/e, F.A. Davis Company, Philadelphia, PA, 1995.

Benson, Michael D. *Obstetrical Pearls: A Practical Guide for the Efficient Resident,* 1/e, F.A. Davis Company, Philadelphia, PA, 1995.

Blackbourne, Lorne H. *Surgical Recall,* 2/e, William and Wilkins, Baltimore, MD, 1998.

Callahan, Tamara L., et al. *Blueprints in Obstetrics and Gynecology,* 1/e, Blackwell Science, Malden, MA, 1998.

Carey et al. *The Washington Manual of Medical Therapeutics,* 29/e, Lippincott, William and Wilkins, Baltimore, MD, 1998.

Cecil, Russell L., Charles A. Carpenter, Thomas E. Andreoli, J. Claude Bennet, and Fred Plum. *Cecil's Essentials of Medicine*, 4/e, W. B. Saunders Co., Philadelphia, 1997.

Cotran, Ramzi S., Vinay Kumar, and Tucker Collins. *Robbins' Pathologic Basis of Disease,* 6/e, W.B. Saunders Co., Philadelphia, 1999.

Daldah, N.S., N.H. Doesburg, and P. Russo. *Pediatric and Developmental Pathology*, Vol. 5, September 1, 1998.

Dale, C.D. and Daniel D. Federman. *Scientific American Medicine*, Scientific American Inc., http://www.samed.com, 1998.

Dawson-Saunders, Beth and Robert G. Trapp. *Basic and Clinical Biostatistics,* 2/e, Appleton and Lange, Stamford, CT, 1994.

DeCherney, Alan and Martin Pernoll. *Current Obstetric and Gynecologic Diagnosis and Treatment*, 8/e, Appleton and Lange, Stamford, CT, 1994.

Delisa, Joel A., Bruce M. Gaus, and William L. Bockenek. *Rehabilitation Medicine: Principles and Practice,* 3/e, Lippincott-Raven, Baltimore, MD, 1998.

Ewald, Gregory A. and Clark R. McKenzie. *The Washington Manual of Medical Therapeutics,* 28/e, Little, Brown, and Company, 1995.

Farber, E.M. and M.L. Nall. *The Natural History of Psoriasis in 5,600 Patients*, Dermatologica; Vol. 148, 1974.

Fauci, Anthony S., et al. *Harrison's Principles of Internal Medicine,* 13/e, McGraw-Hill, New York, 1994.

Fauci, Anthony S., et al. *Harrison's Principles of Internal Medicine,* 14/e, McGraw-Hill, New York, 1998.

Ferri, Fred F. *Practical Guide to the Care of the Medical Patient,* 3/e, Mosby-Year Book, St. Louis, MI, 1995.

Friedman, Gary D. *Primer of Epidemiology*, 4/e, McGraw-Hill, New York, 1994.

Friedman, Harold H. *Problem-Oriented Medical Diagnosis,* 6/e, Lippincott, William and Wilkins, Baltimore, MD, 1996.

Gabbard, Glenn O. *Treatments of Psychiatric Disorders*, American Psychiatric Press Inc., 1995.

Greenberg, R.S., S.R. Daniels, W.D. Flanders, J.W. Eley, and J.R. Boring. *Medical Epidemiology*, 2/e, Appleton and Lange, East Norwalk, CT, 1996.

Goldman, Howard. *Review of General Psychiatry*, 4/e, Appleton and Lange, East Norwalk, CT, 1995.

Gorbach, Sherwood L., John G. Bartlett, Richard Zorab and Neil R. Blacklow. *Infectious Diseases*, 2/e, W.B. Saunders Co., Philadelphia, 1997.

Goroll, Allan H., Lawrence A. May, and Albert G. Mulley, Jr. *Primary Care Medicine: Office Evaluation and Management of the Adult Patient,* 3/e, Lippincott-Raven Publishers, Philadelphia, 1995.

Hakker, Neville and J. George Moore. *Essentials of Obstetrics and Gynecology*, 2/e, W.B. Saunders Co., Philadelphia, 1992.

Hall and Ellman. *Heath Care Law and Ethics,* West Publishing Company, 1990.

Hay, William W., Jr., Jessie R. Groothius, and Anthony Hayward. *Current Pediatric Diagnosis & Treatment,* 13/e, Appleton and Lange, Stamford, CT, 1997.

Hay et al. *Current Pediatric Diagnosis & Treatment,* 14/e, Appleton and Lange, Stamford, CT, 1999.

Hoffman, Ronald. *Hematology, Basic Principles and Practice,* 2/e, Churchill Livingston Inc., 1995.

Jarell, Bruce E. and R. Anthony Carabasi. *NMS Surgery,* 2/e, Lippincott, William and Wilkins, Baltimore, MD, 1991.

Jonsen, Albert R., Mark Siegler, William J. Winslade, and Mark Seigler. *Clinical Ethics: A Practical Approach to Ethical Decisions in Clinical Medicine*, 4/e, McGraw-Hill, New York, 1997.

Kaplan, Harold I. And Benjamin J. Sadock. *Comprehensive Textbook of Psychiatry,* 7/e, Williams and Wilkins, Baltimore, MD, 1997.

Kaplan, Harold I. and Benjamin J. Sadock. *Kaplan and Sadock's Synopsis of Psychiatry: Behavioral Sciences/Clinical Psychiatry,* 8/e, Lippincott, Williams, and Wilkins, Baltimore, MD, 1998.

Katzung, Bertram G. *Basic and Clinical Pharmacology*, 7/e, Appleton and Lange, Stamford, CT, 1998.

Levinson, Warren E. and Ernest Jawetz. *Medical Microbiology and Immunology,* 3/e, Appleton and Lange, East Norwalk, CT, 1994.

MacLeod, Carter and A.P.M. Forest. *Principles and Practice of Surgery*, Churchill Livingstone, 1990.

Marino, Bradley. *Blueprints in Pediatrics,* 1/e, Blackwell Science, Malden, MA, 1998.

Markovchick, Vincent J. and Peter T. Pons. *Emergency Medicine Secrets,* 2/e, Hanley and Belfus. 1993.

Merenstein, Gerald B., David W. Kaplan, and Adam A. Rosenberg. *Handbook of Pediatrics,* 18/e, Appleton and Lange, Stamford, CT, 1997.

Murphy, Michael J. et al. *Blueprints in Psychiatry,* 1/e, Blackwell Science, Malden, MA, 1997.

Mycek, Mary Julia, Richard A. Harvey, and Pamela C. Champe. *Lippincott's Pharmacology*, 2/e, Lippincott, Williams, and Wilkins, Baltimore, MD, 1997.

Nelson, Waldo E., Richard E. Behrman, and Robert M. Kliegman. *Nelson Essentials of Pediatrics,* 3/e, W.B. Saunders Co., Philadelphia, 1998.

Nicol, Diana, Stephen J. McPhee, and Tony M. Chou. *Pocket Guide to Diagnostic Tests,* 2/e, Appleton and Lange, Stamford, CT, 1996.

Novelline, Robert A. and Lucy Frank. *Squire's Fundamentals of Radiology,* 5/e, Harvard University Press, Cambridge, MA, 1997.

Pansky, Ben. *Review of Gross Anatomy*, 6/e, McGraw-Hill, New York, 1995.
Rambo, William M. *The Student's Textbook of Surgery,* Blackwell Science, Malden, MA, 1996.

Ritchie, Wallace P., Jr., Glenn Steele, Jr., and Richard H. Dean. *General Surgery*, Lippincott Company, 1995.

Schwartz, George R. *Principles and Practice of Emergency Medicine,* 4/e, Lippincott, Williams, and Wilkins, Baltimore, MD, 1998.

Scott, James R., Philip J. Disaia, and Charles B. Hammond. *Danforth's Obstetrics and Gynecology,* 7/e, Lippincott Williams & Wilkins Publishers, Baltimore, MD, 1998.

Speroff, Leon, Robert H. Glass, and Nathan G. Kase. *Clinical Gynecologic Endocrinology and Infertility,* 5/e, Lippincott Williams & Wilkins Publishers, Baltimore, MD, 1995.

Tierney, Lawrence M., Jr., et al. *Current Medical Diagnosis and Treatment,* 38/e, Appleton and Lange, Stamford, CT, 1999.

du Vivier, Anthony and Phillip McKee. *Atlas of Clinical Dermatology,* 2/e, Gower Medical Publishing, 1992.

Way, Lawrence W. *Current Surgical Diagnosis and Treatment,* 10/e, Appleton & Lange, East Norwalk, CT, 1994.

All About the Stanford Solutions Team

Scott J. Kush is a medical/law student who is interested in emergency medicine and venture capitalism. As well as running Planet Med Publishing, he is also becoming actively involved with Silicon Valley start-ups and biotechnology. Recently, he has been working with information technology to create highly interactive tools for medical education.

Tessa L. Walters graduated with her MD from Stanford in 1999 and will start a residency in internal medicine in June 2000. A native of southern California, she is spending another year in the sun at Stanford studying novel biowarfare defenses as a postdoctoral fellow at the Center for International Security and Cooperation. Her interests include international travel, snorkelling, volleyball and eating at innovative restaurants.

Devon J. Webster received her MD from Stanford in 1999 and began a residency in Internal Medicine. Medical interests include stem cell gene therapy, critical care ethics, and gay and lesbian health care. Outside the hospital she enjoys leading a cappella groups, two-stepping, and making very complicated Halloween costumes.

Roni Zeiger received his MD from Stanford and began a residency in internal medicine at UCSF in 1999. A native of Chile, his interests include language barriers in medicine, riding his bicycle, and eating good food with his girlfriend. He plans to practice and teach clinical medicine.

Niaz Banaiee is a medical student who is interested infectious diseases. He is a native of Iran and his hobbies include outdoors and traveling.

Lisa Ann Carroll is a fourth year medical student and received a bachelors degree in history from Princeton University in 1996. She is now devoting a full year to wound healing research in the Stanford Otolaryngology Department. She is currently considering a career in dermatology or ENT/facial plastics.

Swaine L. Chen is an MD/PhD student studying the bacterial cell cycle for his doctoral thesis. He enjoys playing volleyball, tennis, and soccer in his free time. After graduation from Stanford in several years, he hopes to pursue a career in biomedical research.

Sujoya Dey is a fourth year medical student who will start an internal medicine residency in 2000. She is interested in cardiology and plans to incorporate clinical research and teaching in her practice. Outside of school, she loves to swim, sing, and spend time with her friends and family.

Amarjit Dosanjh is a third year medical student with an interest in reconstructive surgery. He is currently doing research on the pathobiology of hemangioma formation. Amarjit is finally ready to finish his preclinical work and start clinics.

Shireen Victoria Guide is a fourth year medical student at Stanford University, currently on a Med Scholars Fellowship doing research on the alpha-6 beta-4 integrin and its implications in cancer, wound healing, and gene therapy. In her spare time, she pursues her passion for the fine arts through salsa and ballroom dancing, singing and playing piano.

George R. Matcuk, Jr. is a second year medical student debating between careers in pediatrics, sports medicine, emergency medicine, or even surgery. He recently decided to do a fifth year of medical school to explore opportunities using computers and to spend more time swimming, running, and hanging out with friends. He thanks his family, especially his father and mother, George and Linda, for their love and support.

Saman Nazarian left Iran 11 years ago and graduated from Stanford Med in 1999. He now spends most of his time in an internal medicine residency at Brigham and Women's Hostpial. In his free time he likes to swim, scuba dive and watch star trek reruns.

Mychelle L. Shegog was born and raised in Cincinnati, Ohio and graduated from Harvard-Radcliffe in 1992. She spent two years working at a health care consulting firm in New York before arriving at Stanford for medical school. She graduated in June of 1999 and has now entered a residency in orthopedic surgery.

Notes

Notes